HUMAN LUNG CANCER RISKS FROM RADON

HUMAN LUNG CANCER RISKS FROM RADON

INFLUENCE FROM BYSTANDER AND ADAPTIVE RESPONSE NON-LINEAR DOSE RESPONSE EFFECTS

Bobby E. Leonard, PhD

International Academy of Hi-Tech Services, Inc.
1007 Rosslare Ct. Arnold, MD 21012

Published by International Academy of Hi-Tech Service, Inc.

1007 Rosslare Ct.

Arnold, MD 21012

FIRST EDITION

Human Lung Cancer Risk From Radon: Influence From Bystander and Adaptive Response Non-Linear Dose Response Effects /

Bobby E. Leonard

ISBN-13: 978-1478116967

ISBN-10: 147811696X

Lung cancer, Radon, Non-Linear Dose Response, Bystander Effects, Adaptive Response Protection

I dedicate this book to Georgia Carol Beecher and my daughter Renee.

CONTENTS

LIST OF TABLES

LIST OF FIGURES

Preface

BEIR VI (1999) eluded to the prospect that future research would uncover radon – lung cancer correlations that could change the outlook relative to the degree of hazard radon imposes to human lung cancer. New research technology developed from the 1980s to 2000, suggested that a federally funded low dose and dose rate radiation effects program was not only warranted but imperative. Congress agreed and $200 million in federal funds were appropriated for a 10 year DOE Low Dose and Dose Rate Research Program in 1999. Morgan (2006) suggested that the newly studied Bystander and Adaptive Response effects will play dominant roles in modeling of non-linear dose response from ionizing radiation. Prior to 1984, radon was considered a health hazard only to uranium miners, when a nuclear worker at the Limerick Nuclear Plant in Pennslyvania set off the plants low level personnel radiation safety monitors. It was found that his home was located over a geological fault where large amounts of radon was escaping. There are now conclusive facts about radon primarily generated by the DOE sponsored research. This text shows the large volume of evidence that Adaptive Response radio-protection (AR), of from 50 to 80%, occurs from single low LET radiation produced charged particle traversals through individual cells. This protection lasts through at least one cell mitotic cycle. Several experiments have shown that the AR protection of low LET radiation is extended to alpha particle cellular damage and should extend to radon alpha particle lung damage. Finally, some of the new case-control studies show zero and negative human lung cancer risks suggesting that they reflect AR protection behavior or that case-control studies provide misleading or erroneous risk results, contrary to the premise of BEIR VI (1999) in their graphical risk Figure 3-2. The endeavor here is to apply microdose analytical techniques to the wealth of dose response data, supportive mainly from a vast amount of published works from the DOE program, to further understand these data and obtain a best understanding of Bystander and Adaptive Response influence on human lung cancer risk from radon.

Relative to the text of this manuscript, the three sections (Chapter 2 – Part I, Chapter 3 – Part II and Chapter 4 – Part III) reporting examination of Bystander Effects, Adaptive Response and Bystander Effects and case- control studies, are structured in the standard research formulation i.e. Introduction, Materials and Method, Results, and Analysis as were the Dose-Response Journal papers (Leonard et al 2011a, 2011b, 2012).

Acknowledgement

This author greatly appreciates the early assistance of Dr. Arthur Lucas of Oklahoma State University in the experimental studies in the test chamber resulting in the measurements of the dynamic behavior of radon progeny (Leonard 1996, 2000) and Andrea George for permitting the measurement of progeny airborne diameters at the US Environment Measurements Laboratory. Gratitude is extended Drs. Leslie Redpath and Edwardo Azzam for discussions relative to their Adaptive Response laboratory measurements that assisted in developing the Microdose Models. The formulation of their Bystander BaD Model by Drs. David Brenner and R. K. Sachs enabled the composite Bystander and Adaptive Response Microdose Model (Leonard 2008a, 2008b) to be developed. Of great significance is the work and discussions with Dr. Ludwig Feinendegen relative to microdosimetry and the use of some of his works. The review by Dr. Ted Rockwell helped in the manuscript productions for the Dose-Response Journal papers. Dr. Richard Thompsons paper on the radon lung cancer risks in Worcester MA motivated the analysis of the case-control studies. His independent statistical analysis of the data with polynomials was supportive of the final conclusions obtained herein. The editing by Ms. Georgia Beecher enabled the voluminous amount of information to be manageable. Finally, thanks is given to Dr. Richard McElroy for assistance in assembling the work into the text presented herein.

Chapter 1 - INTRODUCTORY EXECUTIVE SUMMARY

The National Academy of Science BEIR VI (1999) report estimates 15,400 to 21,800 radon related lung cancer deaths annually in the US. A subsequent EPA (2003) report estimates even higher annual deaths from radon and an uncertainty range from 8,000 to 45,000 thus approaching the annual death rate from motor vehicles. Since the publication of the BEIR VI (1999) report "Health Effects from Exposure to Radon", a significant amount of new data has been published showing various mechanisms that may affect the ultimate assessment of radon as a lung carcinogen, at low domestic and workplace radon levels, in particular, the Bystander Effect and the Adaptive Response radio-protection (AR). The BEIR VI and EPA conclusions relied heavily on human lung cancer case-control studies (see Figure 3-2 of BEIR VI and Figure 1C herein). Since BEIR VI, a number of case-control studies are reported that show a very large variation in human lung cancer risks from radon, which could be affected by BE and AR. The Bystander Effect has principally been observed from the exposure of high LET radiations such as radon progeny emitted alpha particles and has been shown to be absent for low LET radiations such as X-rays, gamma rays and beta particles. Conversely, the Adaptive Response radio-protective effect has been primarily observed for these low LET radiations. If the Adaptive Response protection is affording a protective reduction in the annual radon lung cancer death rate then far more annual lung cancer deaths perhaps should be attributed to cigarette smoking. This manuscript is an extension and consolidation of the work reported earlier in the Dose-Response Journal (Leonard et al 2011a, 2011b, 2012). As was done there, in this manuscript, divided into three parts, we first in Chapter 2 - Part I examine the dose response effect of *in vitro* cell populations from the Bystander Effect induced primarily by radon comparable alpha particles in the absence of low LET radiation.. We analyzed the microbeam and broadbeam alpha particle data of Miller et al (1995, 1999), Zhou et al (2001, 2003, 2004), Nagasawa and Little (1999, 2002), Hei et al (1999), Sawant et al (2001a) and found that the shape of the cellular response to alphas is relatively independent of cell species and LET of the alphas when analyzed in terms of number of alpha particles traversed within the cells. Further, it is conclusively shown that at residential and workplace radon levels that radon induced lung cancer is from Bystander induced cellular damage whereas underground miners received cellular damage from direct alpha particle traversals. This suggests a greater credence to case-control studies relative to high radon underground miners lung cancer

1

data. The same alpha particle traversal dose response behavior should be true for human lung tissue exposure to radon progeny alpha particles. In the Bystander Damage Region of the alpha particle response, we show that there is a variation of RBE from about 10 to 35 in contrast to a single RBE suggested by Miller et al (1995) and many other investigators. A transition region is observed between the Bystander Damage Region (domestic and workplace level damage) and Direct Damage Region (underground miner level damage) of between one and two microdose alpha particle traversals indicating that perhaps two alpha particle "hits" are necessary to produce the direct damage. This was first suggested by Miller et al (1999). Part I also indicates, due to this distinction in types of DNA damage (Ward 1985, 1988, 1995), that extrapolation of underground miners lung cancer risks to human risks at domestic and workplace levels may not be valid.

Recent microdosimetry work for a number of cell species, shows that single (i.e. just one) charged particle traversals through the cell nucleus can activate AR protection. We have, in Chapter 3 - Part II, conducted an analysis based on what is presently known about Adaptive Response and the Bystander Effect and what new research is needed that can assist in the further evaluation human cancer risks from radon. We find, at the UNSCEAR worldwide average human exposures from natural background and man-made radiations, that the human lung receives about a 25% Adaptive Response protection against the radon alpha Bystander damage. At the UNSCEAR minimum range of background exposure levels, the lung receives minimal AR protection but at higher background levels, in the high UNSCEAR range, the lung receives essentially 100% protection from both the radon alpha damage and also the spontaneously occurring, potentially carcinogenic, lung cellular damage.

In Chapter 4 - Part III, we examine case-control studies of human lung cancer risks. These studies compare lung cancer incidences of cohorts exposed to given levels of radon concentrations to non-cancer cohorts under similar living environments. BEIR VI (1999) relied heavily on the case-control studies of relative lung cancer risks from radon. In fact in their summary Relative Risk graph Figure 3-2, over 50% of the lung cancer risk data points in the graph are from case-control studies. As noted above, since the publication of the BEIR VI (1999) report, a significant amount of new case-control data has been published showing a very large variation in lung cancer risks from radon. In Chapter 3 – Part II, it is shown that a very wide range of Adaptive Response radio-protection to humans can occur from natural background and man-made radiations. The case-control radon lung cancer risk data of the new pooled 13 European countries radon study (Darby et al 2005, 2006) and the new 8 North American pooled study (Krewski et al 2005, 2006) have been evaluated in Chapter 4 - Part III. These data comprise a total of 11,746 cases and 20,242 controls. Using the well-known Papworth Poisson Validation Test and a second NETA Poisson Test, it is shown that a single mechanism such as a single linear dose response for human radon induced lung cancer is Poissonly over-dispersed and must be considered invalid. The large variation in the case-control studies odds ratios of lung cancer from radon risk is reconciled, based on the large variation in geological and ecological conditions affecting low LET background radiation levels and variation in the degree of Adaptive Response radio-protection against the Bystander Effect induced lung damage. The analysis clearly shows Bystander Effect radon lung cancer induction and Adaptive Response reduction in lung cancer in some geographical regions is the only valid explanation for the variation in case-control study results. It is estimated that for radon levels up to about 400 Bq m^{-3} there is about a 30% probability that no human lung cancer risk from radon will be experienced and a 20% probability that the risk is below the zero-radon, endogenic spontaneous or perhaps even genetically inheritable lung cancer risk rate. The BEIR VI (1999) and EPA (2003) estimates of human lung cancer deaths from radon are most likely significantly excessive and far more lung cancer deaths should be attributed to smoking. Again the assumption of linearity of human lung cancer risks from radon, by the Linear No-Threshold Model, with increasing radon exposure is invalid.

The Linear No-Threshold Hypothesis as the Conventional Model for Human Dose Response to Ionizing Radiations

Soon after the perfection of the X-ray machine by Wilhelm Roentgen and the isolation of the naturally radioactive element Radium by Marie and Pierre Curie, it was realized that ionizing radiation can cause solid malignant tumors. It was also found that these sources of radiation can, in some instances, provide a cure for solid tumor cancers by the radiations cell killing properties. England, France and Sweden became the early leaders in radio-therapy cancer treatment. Due to radiations harmful aspects, various radiation related agencies were established, and still exist, to recommend and set exposure limit standards [i.e. the International Commission on Radiological Protection (ICRP) and the United States (US) National Council on Radiation Protection and

Measurements (NCRP)] and to formulate radiation quantities, units and measurement standards [i.e. the International Commission on Radiation Units and Measurements (ICRU)]. As more was learned about radiation effects, the recommended exposure limits were, for some period of time, in a state of steady reduction. In the US, first the Atomic Energy Commission regulated occupation exposures and now the Nuclear Regulatory Commission sets the exposure dose equivalent limits for nuclear workers at 5 mSv (1 mSv = 1 milli-Severt = 1 Rem) per annum. Primarily from radiobiology studies and the use of radiation in cancer therapy, it was early hypothesized that the deleterious effects of ionizing radiations varied linearly with tissue dose. This linear hypothesis has been re-inforced into a Linear No-Threshold hypothesis (LNT), based primarily on the study of the thousands of hjgh level radiation exposed human cohorts from the 1945 Japanese A-bomb events.

Figure 1, Application of Linear Dose Response Modeling

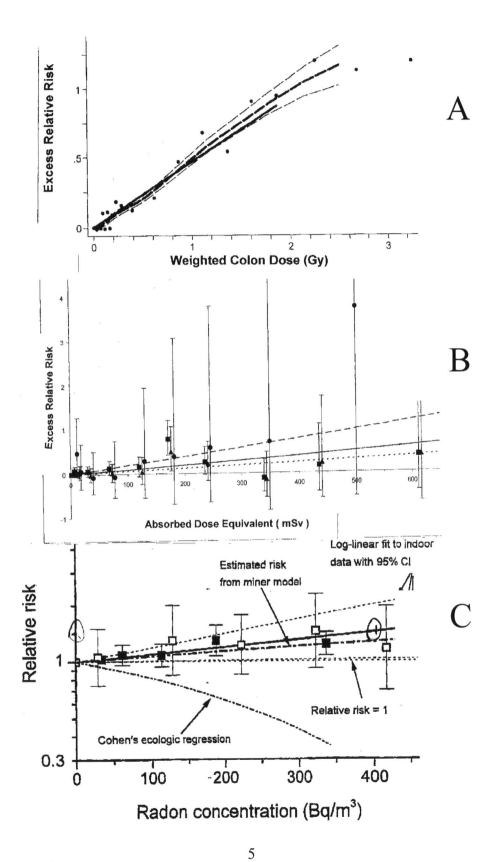

Figure 1 - Application of linear dose response modeling. Panel A – Latest evaluation of radiation risks based on the RERF study of Japanese A-bomb survivors. Excess relative risk of human solid cancers. Reproduced from Preston et al (2007) with permission. The thick solid line is the fitted linear gender-averaged Excess Relative Risk, the thick dashed line is a nonparametric smoothed category-specific estimate and the upper and lower dashed lines are the standard errors. Panel B – Excessive relative risk from 15 country study of nuclear workers for all cancers excluding leukemia; all cancers excluding leukemia, lung and pleural cancers; and leukemia excluding chronic lymphocytic leukemia. Reproduced from Cardis et al (2007) with permission. The solid squares are for all cancers excluding leukemia, the solid diamonds are for all cancers excluding leukemia, lung and pleura and the solid circles are for leukemia excluding chronic lymphocytic leukemia (CCL). The solid line is the ERR best linear fit for all cancers excluding leukemia with slope 0.97 ERR/Sv . Panel C – Summary of relative risks from meta-analysis of indoor-radon studies and from pooled analysis of underground miner studies. The solid squares are data from indoor case-control studies and the open squares are the data from underground miners studies. The thick solid line is the log-linear fit to the indoor data with slope of about 0.0020 ERR/Bq m-3 of radon.Reproduced from BEIR VI (1999) with permission.

.

As Figure 1A, we provide the most recent linear assessment of the Excess Relative Risk (ERR) of Human Solid Cancer Dose Response (Preston et al 2007) based on up-dated Japanese A-bomb survivor data compiled by the specially formed Radiation Effects Research Foundation (RERF). This premise of linearity prevails in almost every study of human dose response to ionizing radiations such as the recent study of the human radiation risks encompassing radiation workers in 15 countries (Cardis et al 2007). We show their Excess Relative Risk data as Figure 1B. During the past 3 decades the US National Academy of Sciences (NAS) National Research Council (NRC) has been evaluating the risks to human health following exposure to ionizing radiation. A series of reports have been issued on biological effects of ionizing radiation beginning with the BEAR I report (BEAR I 1956). Subsequent NAS assessments by committees on the Biological Effects of Ionizing Radiations have been issued as BEIR III (1980), BEIR V (1990) and BEIR VII (2006). It became apparent from the high lung cancer incident rate for underground miners observed in the 1950s and 1960s, that alpha particle emissions to the lung from high levels of radon and its progeny was inducing the lung cancers. Both the US National Academy of Sciences National Research Council and the Environmental Protection Agency (EPA) have evaluated the lung cancer risks from radon. NAS has issued two reports on human health risks for radon and radon progeny exposures also specifying a linearity in dose response, as BEIR IV (1988) and BEIR VI (1999). They also have issued a dosimetry analysis of radon dose response of the underground miners and humans at domestic radon levels (NRC 1991). We noted above that BEIR VI estimates 15,400 to 21,800 radon related lung cancer deaths annually in the US. The recent EPA (2003) report basically is in agreement with the BEIR VI (1999) report

6

findings but provides a higher estimate for annual deaths from radon induced lung cancers. Figure 1C provides the summary of Relative Risks (RR) from Figure 3-2 of the BEIR VI (1999) report. The BEIR VI committee stated that "the choice was to use a linear relationship between risk and low doses of radon progeny without a threshold. The choice was based primarily on considerations related to the stochastic nature of the energy deposition by alpha particles; at low doses, a decrease in dose simply results in a decrease in the number of cells subjected to the same insult. That observation, combined with the evidence that a single alpha particle can cause substantial permanent damage to a cell and that most cancers are of monoclonal origin, provides the mechanistic basis of the use of a linear model at low doses. In addition, as discussed in the report, exposure-response relationships estimated from the observational data in miners with low exposures, and from the case-control studies of indoor radon, are consistent with linearity." The tendency for assumption of linearity has prevailed in the most recent case-control studies and two recent European (Darby et al 2005, 2006) and North American (Krewski et al 2005, 2006) pooled studies. Their jointly stated premise is "That pooling of data from these studies is based on the assumption that between-site differences seen in the observed relationship between lung cancer risk and radon exposure are due to random measurement variability and the true relationship is independent of site locality and only dependent on the carcinogenic sensitivity of human lung tissue to alpha radiation." We show their linearized dose response estimates as Figures 2A and 2B (Linear No-Threshold assumption).

Figure 2, Linear fits of individual studies in two pooled case-control radon studies

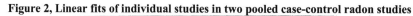

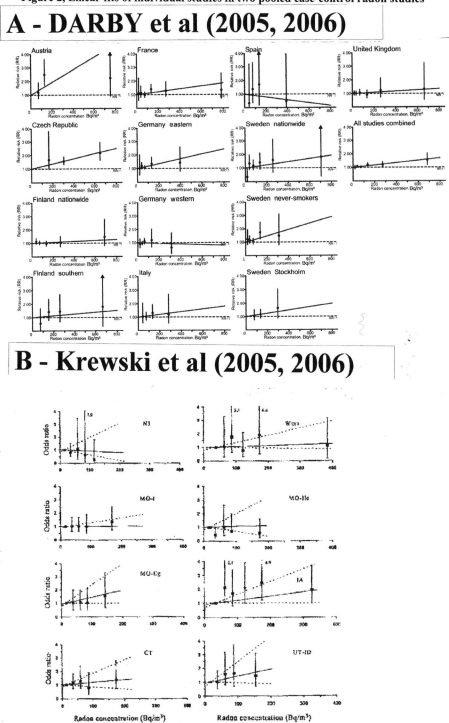

Figure 2 - Linear fits of individual studies in two pooled case-control radon studies. Panel A - Radon relative risks for 13 pooled European case-control studies. From Darby et al (2005, 2006) with permission. Panel B – Radon relative risks for 8 pooled North American case-control studies. From Krewski et al (2005, 2006) with permission.

BEIR VI Dose Response for Human Lung Cancer Risks from Radon and its Progeny

Some prior low LET, alpha particle and specifically radon alpha dose response and "hit" probability data based on biodosimetry studies of organs and systems are cited in BEIR VI (1999). Jostes et al (1993), using the single-cell gel technique, measured cell "hit" probabilities for Chinese hamster and A_L cells from unirradiated, and x-ray and radon alpha exposures showing a Poisson distributed "hit" probability. Brooks et al (1994) measured the effectiveness of radon with respect to ^{60}Co radiations for the induction of micronuclei in rat lung fibroblast (RLF) and Chinese ovary cells in both *in vitro* and *in vivo* (live male Wistar rats). Linear dose responses were estimated. For both *in vitro* and *in vivo*, a Relative Biological Effectiveness of 10.6 ± 1.0 was obtained between radon and ^{60}Co in rat lung fibroblasts. In one of the first reported microbeam alpha particle irradiations, Nelson et al (1996) reported use of the Pacific Northwest Laboratories microbeam facility to irradiate CHO-K1 cells to specific numbers of 3.2 MeV alpha particles. It was found that single alpha particle cell traversals produce micronuclei. The dose response was estimated to be linear for a range from single traversals to five traversals. Significant was the observation that with increased numbers of alpha particles there was a decrease in the ratio of binucleated to mononucleated cells of 3.5% per hit, suggesting that alpha particles induced dose-dependent, Adaptive Response type protective, mitotic delay. Also, since no dose response exposures were below one alpha particle per cell, no Bystander Effects could be expected. Mitchel et al (1999, 2002, 2003), Mitchel (2006, 2007a, 2007b, 2008) have shown Adaptive Response type protection for a number of organs and systems. These will be discussed in Part II and Part III Chapters 3 and 4. Directly related to dose response of the respiratory tract to radon and progeny alpha particles is the work of Brooks et al (1997) where they applied biological dosimetry. *In vivo* biodosimetry were applied to male Wastar rats exposure to deep lung epithelial cells, deep lung fibroblasts, tracheal epithelial cells and nasal epithelial cells. The relative micronuclei radio-sensitivities were determined and the micronuclei dose responses were estimated to be linear.

9

New Evidence of Non-Linear Human Dose Response Since BEIR VI (1999)

In general, the entire concept of the Linear No-Threshold hypothesis has recently been put into question by a number of significant radiobiology studies. At the 2008 annual meeting of NCRP, the results of an international survey of scientists world-wide was reported (Jenkins-Smith 2008) where 70% of those polled believed that the Linear No-Threshold concept should be modified to express possible non-linearity at the very low doses to which humans are nominally exposed. The Health Physics Society has issued a policy statement to the effect that exposures below 50 mSv per year should be considered irrelevant to human health risks (HPS 2004). The French National Academy of Science has issued guidelines for the French nuclear industry stating that human response to low level radiation exposure should be expected to be non-linear (Tubiana et al 2005, 2006, 2007). Even BEIR VII (2006) cites the two independent measurements of dose response of human lymphocytes from X-rays (Lloyd et al 1988, Pohl-Ruling et al 1992) as only conclusively becoming linear above 20 mGy (see Figure 2-5, BEIR VII 2006).

A 10 year, $200 million US Department of Energy (DOE) Low Dose Radiation Research Program was initiated in 2000 to study the various dose response mechanisms that exist at low doses. Primary mechanisms that have been studied are the potentially deleterious Bystander Effect (BE), the potentially beneficial Adaptive Response (AR) effect, the combined low dose hyper-radiosensitivity (HRS) and high dose induced radio-resistance (IRR) as HRS/IRR, the low LET "inverse" dose rate effect (IDRE), the high LET (alpha particle induced) underground miners "inverse" dose rate effect, genomic instability and apoptosis. In particular, the effect of genomic instability in progeny of irradiated cells is not well understood at present. Morgan (2003a, 2003b) provides assessment of how genomic instability could be a major factor in radiation induced carcinogenesis. Morgan (2006) however suggests that the Bystander Effect and Adaptive Response will play the major roles in the future shape of the dose response curve for ionizing radiations. As of December 2008, the DOE Low Dose Radiation Research Program cites 241 and 230 journal papers on Adaptive Response and Bystander Effect, respectively, published since BEIR VI (1999) was issued. Now over 700 papers have been published on these two subjects.

Using microbeam single cell alpha particle exposures, primarily from the Radiological Research Accelerator Facility at Columbia University (Randers-Pehrson et al 2001), the Tandem Van de Graaff Accelerator at Brookhaven National laboratory (Miller et al 1995) and the Gray Laboratory (Folkard et al 1997) microbeam facilities, the Bystander Effect for alpha particles has been conclusively confirmed (Miller et al 1995, 1999, Zhou et al 2001, 2003, 2004, Nagasawa and Little 1999, 2002, Hei et al 1999, Sawant et al 2001a, 2001b) for a number of cell species. It has also been shown, with a Microdose Model, that single radiation induced low LET charged particle traversals through the cell nucleus provides the Poisson distributed activation of Adaptive Response protection (Leonard 2000, 2005, 2007a, 2007b, 2008a, 2008b, Leonard and Leonard 2008). This conclusion is based on the microdose analysis of a number of low LET dose response studies (Azzam et al 1996, Elmore et al 2005, 2006, 2008, Ko et al 2004, Redpath et al 2001, 2003, Redpath and Antoniono 1998, Shadley and Wiencke 1989, Shadley and Wolff 1987, Shadley et al 1987, Wiencke et al 1986, Wolff et al 1989, 1991) encompassing a wide range of low LET radiations. We shall here, in the Results Section, present the most recent microbeam and broadbeam alpha particle Bystander data. In the later sections, we will examine how the new experimental data and modeling methods developed since BEIR VI (1999) may provide a more cognizant estimate of human lung cancer risks from radon progeny considering the new evidence relative to the Bystander Effect and Adaptive Response radio-protection.

Distinction Between Adaptive Response and the Bystander Effect

To evaluate the potential effects of BE and AR at the microdose level, it is first appropriate to explicitly define Bystander Effect and Adaptive Response for the benefit of our analysis in the following sections and the Chapters 3 and 4, Parts II and III. For consistency, we here repeat our earlier description of BE and AR (Leonard 2008a, 2008b). Relative to the Bystander and Adaptive Response effects, distinction entails the examination of the basic definitions of the BE and AR at the microdosimetry level (ICRU 1983). Dr. Eric Hall, a very early contributor to Bystander Effect research with his group at Columbia University, recently defined (Hall 2003) the Bystander Effect as "the induction of biological effects in cells that are not directly traversed by a charged particle, but are in the close proximity to cells that are." Morgan (2006) provided a similar conventional definition of the Bystander Effect behavior as "those effects occurring in cells that were not hit i.e., not traversed by an ionizing particle, but were neighbors of cells that were irradiated". Investigations have encompassed both deleterious and beneficial results in un-hit cells as Bystander Effect (i.e. Leonard and Leonard 2008).

Adaptive Response, for many, has meant the reduction in the biological effects of large doses of ionizing radiation by activation of cellular protective mechanisms with the prior exposure to low doses of radiation. The prior low dose is usually called the "primer" dose and the subsequent large dose the "challenge" dose. However, more recent work has shown the priming dose can also result in a reduction of endogenic spontaneous, naturally occurring, potentially carcinogenic cellular damage. Azzam et al (1996), Redpath et al (2001) and others have logically considered the spontaneous damage priming dose protection also as Adaptive Response. The AR protection seen in endogenic spontaneously occurring damage of course has far greater human radiation risks implications. In general, the Adaptive Response term currently applies to the protective effects in cells directly hit by the priming radiations. Deleterious damage to cells directly hit has conventionally been called Direct Damage. To get more specific, the fundamental question then becomes, "When does charged particle traversals become classified as protective Bystander?". We would first say that any charged particle traversal to any part of a cell, including the cytoplasm and the nucleus, causing a beneficial effect on that specific cell would be considered Adaptive Response. Then what would we call a biological effect to a cell from a traversal through the adjacent intracellular medium? The medium transfer studies of Mothersill and Seymour (1997) is currently considered a Bystander Effect. In a separate joint paper, Mothersill and Seymour (2005) point out that the Bystander Effect could offer beneficial as well as deleterious influences. For low LET radiations, it has been shown that human HeLa x skin cells exhibit a protective Bystander transformation frequency suppression from exposure to low LET 28 kVp mammogram and 60 kVp diagnostic X-rays (Leonard and Leonard 2008, Redpath et al 2003, Ko et al 2004). Hooker et al (2004) have shown that for inversions in pKZ1 mice spleen *in vivo* that an Adaptive Response protection is afforded when only a small number of cells are hit, which can be interpreted as a Bystander protection based on the above conventional definition of the Bystander Effect. The supernatant transfer experiment of Iyer and Lehnert (2002) for alpha particle exposure has been interpreted as a protective Bystander Effect although one can as easily

12

interpret the results as Adaptive Response protection of alpha particle damage by priming doses to the supernatant medium. Technically however, since the intercellular medium was irradiated and not the cell itself, the effect must be considered a Bystander effect.

Chapter 2 - PART I – RADON LUNG CANCER RISKS - INFLUENCE FROM ALPHA PARTICLE INDUCED BYSTANDER EFFECT

1. INTRODUCTION

A number of radio-biologists have posed the question, "What if the Bystander Effect from radon alpha particles is operative within the human lung and is a major cause of lung cancer?" This has prompted studies to examine the potential magnitude and consequences of the radon produced Bystander Effect in human lung tissue (Little and Wakeford 2001, Little 2004, Brenner and Sachs 2002, 2003, Brenner et at 2001). Based on considerable radio-biology research completed since the issuance of BEIR VI (1999), primarily sponsored by the United States (US) Department of Energy Low Dose Research Program, we here in this chapter as Part I, of this three part study, examine the potential influence of the Bystander Effect on human lung cancer risks from radon. In a separate Chapter 3 - Part II, we then pose a similar question, "What if the human lung tissue is responsive to both the deleterious Bystander Effect and also a beneficial Adaptive Response radio-protection with respect to human lung cancer risk from radon?" In Chapter 4 - Part III, we apply the results of the Part I Bystander Effect analysis and the Part II combined Adaptive Response and Bystander Effect analysis to the case-control studies of Odds Ratio Radon Induced Relative Lung Cancer Risks in North America (9 studies), Europe (13 studies) and China (1 study). In this Part I, we are able to show that the alpha particle traversal dose response for transformation frequency and chromosome aberration cell damage is independent of cell species and LET in the LET range for radon progeny alpha particles when evaluated in terms of alpha particle traversals through the cell. In the radon concentration levels to which humans are exposed in the domestic and workplace environment, we show that the carcinogenic producing lung tissue cellular damage from the alpha particles is predominantly from Bystander Effect chromosome damage. Thus, a representative Bystander Effect dose response shape is obtained for radon exposure at domestic levels and it is premised that the lung cancer risk dose response, depicted in Figure 3-2 of BEIR VI (1999) and Figure 1C herein, should not be linear but concave downward from Bystander Effect cell damage. In the Chapter 4 - Part III of this work we show that analysis of sub-sets of the case-control radon pooled lung cancer risk data of Krewski et al (2006) and Darby et al (2006) is not linear but reflect this concave downward dose response behavior [as predicted by the Brenner et al (2001) BaD Model for the Bystander Effect] and in some instances show that human exposure to increased radon concentrations suggests a protection against lung cancer incidence as some case-control studies exhibit.

2. MATERIALS AND METHODS

2.2 The Brenner et al (2001) BaD Model for Bystander Effect Dose Response Behavior

In the following sections we will provide the Bystander BaD Model of Brenner et al (2001) which will then be used with empirical modifications, in the Results Section, to analyze both microbeam and broadbeam data involving only alpha particle irradiations which would be expected to be absent of any Adaptive Response influences since AR is found to be primarily induced by low LET radiations.

2.2.a Emperically Modified BaD Model Analysis of Alpha Particle Studies Relative to Radon Progeny Dose Response in Humans

As mentioned above, there have been a number of studies of the dose response from both microbeam and broadbeam exposures of human tissue to alpha particles (Miller et al 1995, 1999, Zhou et al 2001, Nagasawa and Little 1999, 2002, Hei et al 1999, Sawant et al 2001a, 2001b). In the Results Section, we present detailed analysis of these data for the purpose of identifying explicit characteristics of alpha particle induced, potentially carcinogenic, cellular damage as they impact on the human health risks from radon. It has been an *a priori* assumption that both Bystander Damage and Direct Damage from radon and progeny alpha particles cause human lung cancers. To adequately anticipate human risk, there is the need for evaluating broadbeam *in vivo* exposure responses (a whole body exposure as received by a nuclear worker would be considered " broadbeam") experienced by human exposures by extrapolation from the microbeam *in vitro* data. Brenner et al. (2001) – (see their Figure 3a) – have made a direct comparison of the Bystander Effect between single-cell microbeam and broadbeam cell population exposures *in vitro*. Fundamentally, there is a distinction between microbeam and broadbeam exposures. For microbeam *in vitro* exposures, exact numbers of alpha particles are injected into the cell population, one cell at a time. Then if all the cell population has received at least one microbeam alpha injection, there is no chance of Bystander Effect damage based on the above cited definition of the Bystander Effect. For broadbeam *in vitro* or *in vivo* exposures, the alpha particle traversals are Poisson distributed such that there is a distribution of alpha particle traversals around a Poisson distributed mean number of traversals. Thus, some cells may have zero alpha traversals (and thus subject to Bystander Effect cell damage alone) and some cells with traversals much greater than the mean based on Poisson statistics. Brenner et al (2001) have thus modeled the dose response behavior for the Bystander Effect for both single-particle (microbeam) *in vitro* and what may be predicted for Poisson distributed particle broadbeam exposures *in vivo* and *in vitro* laboratory exposures. From Equation (9) of Brenner et al (2001), we provide the BaD Model equation for microbeam exposures given, for transformation frequency TF, by

$$TF = f \gamma N q^N + (1 - f) \sigma F(N) \qquad (1)$$

f is the fraction of cells hit by microbeam alpha particles, N is the exact number of hits per cell, q is the probability of a cell surviving a single alpha particle traversal of its nucleus, γ then is the direct damage production rate of oncogenic transformations per surviving cell that has experienced an alpha particle traversal. σ = the fraction of cells that are hypersensitive to oncogenic transformation (or prevention of transformations for protective Bystander mechanisms, in which case use of a negative σ would be required, but not to imply a negative population of cells only that the hypersensitivity produces a negative response which could be for example from the reduction of natural, spontaneous damage). F(N) is the Bystander killing term. In the case of the Sawant et al (2001a, 2001b) exposures represented by Equation (9) of Brenner et al (2001), f = 0.1 or 1 in 10 cells. There is no term for the spontaneous transformation frequency in the present microbeam BaD Model or the broadbeam BaD model given below. Little and Wakeford (2001) added a constant spontaneous term in their examination of radon induced lung cancer [see their Equation (4)]. A simplified version for the Brenner et al (2001) broadbeam, BaD Model [see their Equation (13)], relation is

$$TF = \gamma q <N> + \sigma [1 - \exp(-k <N>)] \exp(-q <N>) \qquad (2)$$

16

Figure 3, Illustration of the bystander BaD

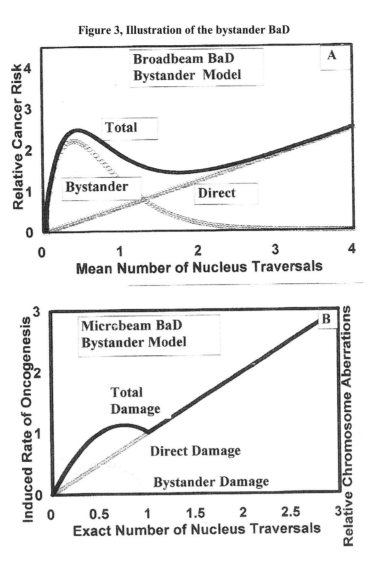

Figure 3 - Illustration of the bystander BaD Model showing bystander and direct cellular damage (Brenner et al 2001). Panel A – Broadbeam. Panel B – Microbeam.

As Figure 3A, we provide a reproduction of their Figure 4 illustration of the broadbeam BaD Bystander model given by Equation (2) for broadbeam exposures. Page 259 of Hall (2000) provides a description of the methods for transformation frequency analysis. Brenner et al (2001) define γq as the slope of the direct damage dose response for oncogenic transformation for a Poisson distributed mean number of alpha particle traversals $<N>$ and thus is the direct damage oncogenic transformation production rate per mean alpha particle traversal, In Equation (2), $<N>$ is the Poisson distributed mean number of alpha particle nucleus traversals and k is the number of the unirradiated neighbor cells that receive a Bystander responsive signal (Brenner et al 2001). The first term in Equations (1) and (2) is the linear direct damage term as shown in Figure 3. As noted by Brenner et al (2001), since <N> is proportional to dose [in our composite model (Leonard 2008a), which was applied to *in vitro* broadbeam exposures, we have included both linear and quadratic direct damage although at low doses the behavior is primarily linear], this corresponds to the α D linear term in the conventional linear-quadratic dose response equation (Kellerer and Rossi 1972). The second term in Equations (1) and (2) is the Bystander damage contribution to the transformation frequency. Brenner et al (2001) proposes that the Bystander Effect is as a result of a small population of hypersensitive Bystander receptor cells such that the [exp (- q <N>)] "Depletion" transition function in Equation (2) characterizes the depletion of these hypersensitive cells by inactivation by hits from the direct damage. The [1- exp (- k <N>)] "Hit probability" transition function provides the probability that at least one cell is directly hit where, as noted, k is the number of unirradiated neighbor cells receiving the Bystander signal. In Figure 3A, we show how these two functions behave with increased dose (and alpha charged particle track traversals) and combine as the product [1- exp (- k <N>)] [exp (- q <N>)] to facilitate the total Bystander Damage component of broadbeam BaD Model. As noted above, this broadbeam BaD Model Equation (2) has been applied to high LET radon dose response (Little and Wakeford 2001, Brenner et al 2001, Little 2004, Brenner and Sachs 2002). In earlier work, we have used the empirically modified BaD Model to examine Bystander behavior for the broadbeam alpha particle data of Miller et al (1999) and Nagasawa and Little (1999) [see Figure 7a and 7b, Leonard (2007a)]   In section 3.1.b below, we show the analysis of the microbeam human-hamster hybrid (CHO K1) exposure data of Hei et al (1999) and Zhou et al (2001) for low exposures (hits) of 5, 10, 20 and 100% (as well as 1, 2, 4 and 8 exact hits to 100%) of the cell populations. Other work has shown that the range of the Bystander signal in tissue is approximately 210 μm (Leonard 2009, Belyakov et al 2005) and the diameter of CHO cells approximately 12.5 μm (Jostes et al 1993) such that, for those percentages, Equation (2) may be used to compare the Hei et al (1999) and Zhou et al (2001) data in Section 3.1.b with the Nagasawa and Little (1999) data in Section 3.1.c as far as Bystander and Direct Damage response. Further, we have noted above that in the Poisson distributed broadbeam exposures, the Poisson distribution will predict a finite number of cells in any population that receives no alpha traversals. This is why the depletion function is exponential in behavior in Equation (2), accounting for the "residual" non-hit cells for greater than a mean cell hits of unity i.e. $<N> \geq 1.0$. Here as was true for others (Little and Wakeford 2001, Brenner et al 2001, Little 2004, Brenner and Sachs 2002) we have used the cell nucleus as the sensitive volume. The mean number of nucleus traversals can be approximated by the division of the tissue absorbed dose in cGy by the specific energy deposited per nucleus traversal (hits per cGy), $<z1>$ (assuming a contiguous cell population) [see Equation (4) Section 2.3.b].

In the special case for microbeam exposures where fractions, f, of the cell population are injected with equal number of alpha particles, we can write the microbeam Equation

$$TF = f \gamma q^N + (1- f) \sigma [1- Exp (- k' N)] \text{ for } f < 1.0$$
$$\text{and } TF = \gamma q^N \quad \text{for } f \geq 1.0 \tag{3}$$

We see that the second, Bystander term becomes zero when 100% of cells are hit based on the premise by Brenner et al (2001) that a directly hit cell becomes insensitive to the Bystander effect. Figure 3B illustrates this case. Appendix B provides explicit definitions for the parameters for the empirically modified BaD Model.

2.3 The Human Lung Cells as "Targets" for High and Low LET Traversals and Subsequent Energy Depositions per Traversal

It is recognized that the traversal of radiation induced charged particles (hits) to exposed cells involves the microscopic statistical accumulation of these hits. In particular, Kellerer and Rossi (1972), Bond et al (1985), Varma et al (1981), ICRU Report 36 (ICRU 1983) and Rossi and Zaider (1996) have greatly contributed to the basic microdosimetry concepts of tissue micromass, a microdose, the stochastic specific energy deposition, z_1, and the fluence derived non-stochastic quantity mean Specific Energy Deposition per Charged Particle Traversal (hit), $<z_1>$ used in our modeling here. We respectfully refer to the Leonard (2007a) sections "Energy depositions and activation of response events at very low doses at the microscopic level", "A Poisson distributed accumulation threshold function" and Figure 1 (Regarding the Poisson function provides the distribution for "at least 1 hit", "at least 2 hits", "at least 3 hits", etc.) in the Materials and Methods Section therein.

2.3.a *The Size of the Human Lung Target Cells Susceptible to Carcinogenesis*

Simmons and Richards (1988) provide the volume of the human lung cell to be 78 μm^3 using an image analyzer. Obviously, since there are three human lung cell species that are known to be sensitive to radon induced lung cancer i.e. bronchial basal, bronchial secretory and Bronchiolar Secretory (BEIR VI 1999, NRC 1991), it is naive to suggest a single representative lung cell diameter for lung cancer studies. It is well known that even for a given cell species within a given tissue there is a wide variation in size. Others have found that these three human lung cell types each vary in size and hence present different target sizes for radiation microdose "Hits" from the radon progeny alpha particles and the low LET AR inducing radiations. Table 2-1 of BEIR VI (1999) shows that the bronchial secretory cells are much larger in diameter than the bronchial basal cells. Little and Wakeford (2001) used these data to estimate annual lung cell "Hit" rates per Bq m^{-3} of radon. Brenner and Sachs (2002) uses a cell cross-section area of 25 μm^2 for the bronchial basal cell nucleus and notes that a radon concentration of 100 Bq m^{-3} produces 0.3 alpha particle traversals in 60 years of exposure. From these numbers, for our analysis we estimate the three cell diameters to be 9.0, 17.7 and 10.7 μm for the bronchial basal, bronchial secretory and the bronchiolar secretory cells, respectively. These are for flattened, spheroid shaped *in vitro* cell measurements. These are in agreement with the BEIR VI (1999) Table 2-1 data and the same data used by Little and Wakeford (2001). We use these diameters in Table A1, A2 and A3 of Appendix A of Part II to estimate the Specific Energy Deposition per Nucleus Traversals for the low LET radiations received by the lung from human exposures at the UNSCEAR (2000) world average low LET human exposure levels.

2.3.b *Method for Determination of the Mean Specific Energy per Sensitive Volume Hit - < z_1 >*

The amount of radiation energy deposited, on a microdose level, into the cells sensitive volume by a charged particle traversal is dependent on the dose-averaged linear energy transfer, $\bar{L}_D$ (in units of keV / micrometer) and the mean chord length, ℓ (in units of μm), traversed through the sensitive volume. As was the case in the earlier works (Leonard 2005, 2007a, 2007b, 2008a, 2008b, Leonard and Leonard 2008) the sensitive volume here is chosen to be the nucleus for the three human lung cell species, based on the microbeam measurements by Miller et al (1999) where it was found that the cytoplasm is insensitive to alpha particle traversals. Others have suggested that the cytoplasm is also sensitive to Bystander responses (Shao et al 2004, Wu et al 1999). In all our AR Microdose Model examinations use of the nucleus has been found to provide the best fit of the model to the empirical data. BEIR VI (1999) and James et al (2004) in their analysis with respect to alpha particle traversals consider the nucleus as the sensitive region for lung cancer induction. The dose-averaged LET of the radiation in tissue and chord length traversed provides the energy deposited into the sensitive volume per traversal (Hit). Absorbed dose is energy deposited per unit mass of tissue. Knowing the diameter of the sensitive volume, the volume and the mass, m(g), of the sensitive volume may be obtained using a mean cell density of 1.04 g cm^{-3} (Attix 1986). This provides the energy deposited per unit mass, $E(keV\ g^{-1}) = \bar{L}_D\ \ell\ /\ m$ for a single charged particle track across the sensitive volume. With the energy to absorbed dose conversion factor (1.6022 x 10^{-11} cGy g keV^{-1}), we have $<z_1> = D(cGy\ per\ hit) = 1.6022$ x 10^{-11} (cGy g keV^{-1}) x $E(keV\ g^{-1}$ per hit). Thus,

$$<z_1> = Dose/Hit\ (track) = 1.6022\ x\ 10^{-11}(cGy\ g\ keV^{-1})\ \bar{L}_D(keV\ \mu m^{-1})\ \ell\ (\mu m)\ m(g)^{-1}\quad (4)$$

Several investigators have examined the chord length problem (Kellerer 1984, Ellett and Braby 1972, Enns and Ehlers 1993). By considering the mean chord length per cell cross-section area, an analytical approximation for $<z_1>$ was offered by Kellerer and Rossi (1972) as a function of spherical critical volume diameter, d, and the dose-averaged linear energy transfer, $\bar{L}_D$, of the radiation, i.e.

$$<z_1> = 22.95(cGy\ g\ keV^{-1}\ /\ chord\ length-\mu m)\ \bar{L}_D\ /\ \rho\ d^2 cGy\ per\ Hit\ (nucleus\ traversal)\quad (5)$$

where ρ = density of cell tissue (see Equation 4.2, Kellerer and Rossi 1972).

We estimate the accuracy in determining the cell nucleus diameters to be about ± 20 %SD, based on direct experience with microscope images and observed variation of cell size. The overall accuracy of $<z_1>$ is thus about ± 30 %SD due to uncertainties in $\bar{L}_D$ also. The impact of this on the use of the model is addressed in Leonard (2008b).

2.3.c New Evidence About the Cellular Sensitive Volume and Alpha Particle Hit Rates for Human Lung Cancer Induction From Radon

A reassessment of the alpha particle dosimetry for the BEIR VI (1999) report has recently been provided by James et al (2004). The important 30 day lung cell mitotic cycle single particle hit probabilities are given in their Table 12 (The three lung cell species that are known to be cancer sensitive are known to have approximately 30 day mitotic cycles.). The ICRP (1994) Report 66 reassessed values as given in James et al (2004) Table 12 are 0.36, 1.4 and 0.51 hits per Basal, Bronchial Secretrory and Bronchiolar Secretory cells respectively per kBq m^{-3} of radon for cell nucleus hits and 1.0, 16, and 4.0 hits per Basal, Bronchial Secretrory and Bronchiolar Secretory cells respectively per kBq m^{-3} of radon for cell cytoplasm hits (entire cell as "target").

Figure 4, The James et al (2004) radon alpha particle hit probabilities

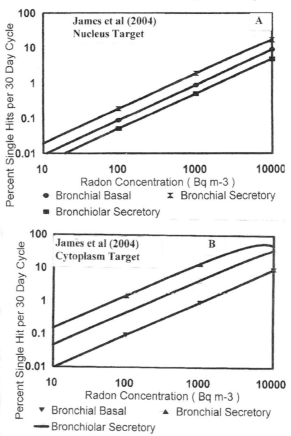

Figure 4 - The James et al (2004) radon alpha particle hit probabilities during the 30 day mitotic cycle for human lung cells. Panel A - bronchial basal and secretory and bronchiolar secretory with cell nucleus as target. Panel B – Same as Panel A, but for cell cytoplasm as target.

As Figure 4 herein, we have provided graphs of the variation in single alpha hit probabilities for the three primarily alpha induced cancer sensitive cells in the lung i.e. as indicated in the legend - the Bronchial Basal, the Bronchial Secretory and the Bronchiolar Secretory cells (James et al 2004).

2.3.d The Emperically Modified BaD Model for Alpha Particle Nucleus Traversals and Dose Response Analysis

To examine the basic properties of broadbeam cellular dose response to alpha particles in the very low dose range, we must include the Bystander and direct damage components encompassed by the Brenner et al (2001) BaD Model. Thus, as a starting point in developing an analytical formulation for the dose response we begin with the BaD Model. Unlike the microbeam BaD Model equation which provides discrete response for intergers of exact numbers of traversals, the broadbeam BaD Model analytical equation provides a continuos function of broadbeam mean number of traversals, $<N>$, derived from the alpha particle exposure fluence and corresponding tissue absorbed dose, D. We showed in Section 2.3.b that D is energy deposited per unit mass of tissue in cGy. For individual cells exposed *in vitro*, Kellerer and Rossi (1972) showed that the amount of energy deposited is proportional to the area of the nucleus. Then the mean number of alpha nucleus traversals is given by

$$\text{Mean Number of Nucleus Traversals} = D / <z_1> \tag{6}$$

Where $<z_1>$ is the specific energy deposition per nucleus traversal (hit), in mean cGy per traversal as defined above. As was the case for low LET charged particle traversals in our Adaptive Response analysis (Leonard 2007a, 2007b), the Poisson distributed mean number of traversals is a continuous function since dose is a continuous function. In Section 4.1.a, the introduction of the Normal Distribution function to fit the transition from Bystander to direct damage experimental data for the mean traversals in that region is non-conventional, unlike the conventional approach where one models the dose-response function using N as the independent variable, then averages the function over the microdose distribution to get a result applicable to broadbeam or radon exposures. We have used the results that have been derived for the broadbeam exposures and then modified these results with the empirical Normal Distribution function to fit the shape of the experimental response. The Normal Distribution function is a continuous

23

function compatible with dose and mean number of traversals but, at present, with no biological meaning.

2.4.a Method - Alpha Particle Dose Response in the Absence of Low LET Adaptive Response Inducing Radiation

We use the emperically modified BaD Microdose Model to examine what has been learned about cellular response to alpha particles, from both microbeam and broadbeam studies. What will be found is that cellular response to only alpha particles (no low LET radiations present) have a specific dose response behavior and, as proposed in the earlier work (Leonard 2008a, 2008b, Leonard and Leonard 2008), there are two distinct regions, a Bystander Damage Region and a Direct Damage Region, exactly as predicted by the Bystander BaD Model presented above and shown in Figure 3. But we also find evidence that there is a threshold and transition dose response region between the Bystander Damage Region and the Direct Damage Region and make an empirical modification to the model.

3. RESULTS

3.1 Examination and Modeling For Alpha Particle microbeam and broadbeam Dose Response Data

We here examine a number of different experimental data sets involving microbeam and broadbeam exposures of different cell species to alpha particle radiation. In particular we use a modified version of the Bystander BaD Model originally provided by Brenner et al (2001) given by Equation (7) below. Through the course of the modeling we have found that the dose response consistently exhibits a threshold for the Direct Damage component. We also find that the high dose Direct Damage behavior is linear-quadratic for both induction of neoplastic transformation (TF) and chromitid and chromotine chromosome aberrations (CA). Thus, these minor modifications, provided by Equation (6), has been made to the basic BaD Model and the composite Adaptive Response and Bystander Microdose Model (Leonard 2008a). We find that the TF and CA data are in agreement that Bystander damage is consistently experienced in the number of cell species studied.

3.1.a Comparison Between Single and Broadbeam Alpha Charged Particle Traversal Induction of Neoplastic Transformation and Chromosome Aberrations

Radiation damage production of neoplastic transformation and chromosome aberrations are believed to be direct indications of ionizing radiations ability to produce carcinogens in human tissue. We use the empirically modified BaD Bystander dose response model of Brenner et al (2001) to analyze alpha particle dose response data provided primarily by Dr. Halls group at Columbia University.

Figure 5, The modified BaD Model best fit to the alpha particle microbeam and broadbeam exposure data

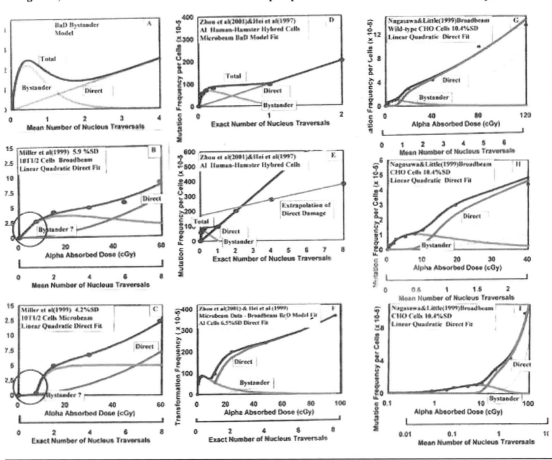

Figure 5 - The modified BaD Model best fit to the alpha particle microbeam and broadbeam exposure data of Miller et al (1999), Zhou et al (2001), Hei et al (1999) and Nagasawa and Little (1999, 2003). Described in Sections 3.1.a, 3.1.b and 3.1.c. Best fit parameter values are given in Table 1.

For direct correlation, we repeat the illustrative BaD Model as Figure 5A. In the experimental data shown in Figures 5B through 5I, we show the transformation frequency as a function of both Alpha Absorbed Dose and microdose alpha particle nucleus traversals. In Figures 5B and 5C as a comparison between broadbeam and microbeam alpha particle response, we present the data of Miller et al (1999) for broadbeam (5B) and microbeam (5C) exposures of C310T1/2 cells to 5.3 MeV alpha particles. For the broadbeam exposures, the alpha fluence was sufficient to deliver a Poisson mean of one alpha particle per cell at the lowest exposure level. In the Figure 5C, they injected exact numbers of alpha particle per cell with the lowest number being one alpha per cell to 100% of the cells. We have not fit the BaD Model parameters to the data, because there are no data in the Bystander dose response region. Since, by definition of Bystander Effect, no data was for less than one traversal, there can be no observed Bystander Effect and thus no values were obtained for the BaD Model parameters σ, ξ, γ, and k in the Table 1 summary of model parameters. We have circled the region between 0 and 1 specific energy hits where BE would be observed, as we will see in the other Figures 5D through 5I given below in Section 3.1.b from other Dr. Halls group data, where exposures were indeed made in the Bystander region. We have fit an empirical function to the data, which, as we will discuss below in Section 4.1.a, suggests a minimal Normal Distribution accumulation of 2 alpha traversals to achieve a quasi-linear-quadratic direct damage response. The idea that more than single hits are necessary to activate the direct damage was first suggested by Miller et al (1999) and here we use the Normal Distribution simply to empirically shape the dose response curve. Other causes such as a reduction in the spontaneous damage level by single hits may be the plausible mechanism. The Normal Distribution function threshold and α and β linear-quadratic parameters to the least squares best fit are given in Table 1. As appropriate, no values for the parameters σ, ξ, γ and k are given.

Table 1, Summary Analysis of Data - Values of Bad Bystander Model

Table. 1 - Summary - Analysis of Data ... - Values of BaD Bystander Model Parameters By Iterative Method of Least Squares for Alpha and Other High LET Particle In Vitro Exposures

Part I -

Investigators	Miller et al (1999)	Miller et al (1999)	Zhou et al (2001))	Nagasawa&Little(1999)	Nagasawa&Little(2002)	
Type Exposure	Micro-beam	Broadbeam	Micro-beam	Broadbeam	Broadbeam	Broadbeam
Radiation	5.3 MeV alphas	5.3 MeV alphas	3.7 MeV alphas	3.7 MeV alphas	3.7 MeV alphas	3.7 MeV alphas
Cells	10T1/2 fibroblast	10T1/2 fibroblast	AL	Wild-type CHO	Wild-type CHO	RepairDeficientxxr-
"Endpoint"	Transformations	Transformations	Transformations	HPRT mutations	Chromosome Aberations	
LET (keV/um)	90	90	112	112	112	112
$<z_1>$ Alpha	7.4	7.4	17.4	17.4	17.4	17.4
Linear-Quadratic Fit %SD	4.2%	5.9 %	6.5%	10.4 %	36.5%	24.6%
BYSTANDER PARAMETERS						
Sigma / Pspon	N/A	N/A	N/A	2.2	1.05	1.05
q (per hit)				1.0	1.0	1.0
k (per hit)				3	2.3	2.3
Zeta				1.0	1.0	1.0
Nu (per hit)	0.07	0.07	1.2	0	0.2	0.2
Beta (per hit2)	0.11	0.1	2.6	0.2	0	0
DirectDamageNormalHits - V	N/A	N/A	N/A	1.5	1.7	1.7
Width Half Maximum - Hits				0.5	0.8	0.8

Part II - All Data From Miller et al (1995) Study of LETs and RBEs for Range of Accelerator High LET Particle Energies

Type Exposure	Broadbeam	Broadbeam	Broadbeam	Broadbeam	Broadbeam	Broadbeam
Radiation	5.00 MeV He-3	5.12 MeV He=4	3.33 MeV He-4	2.37 MeV He-4	1,44 MeV He-3	91.6 MeV F-19
Cells	C3H 10T1/2	C3H 10T1/2	C3H 10T1/2	C3H 10T1/2	C3H 10T1/2	C3H 10T1/2
"Endpoint"	Transformations	Transformations	Transformations	Transformations	Transformations	Transformations
LET (keV/um)	75	90	120	150	200	600
$<z_1>$ Alpha	6.2	7.6	9.9	12.3	16.4	49.3
Linear-Quadratic Fit %SD	4.8%	15.9 %	11.4%	12.1%	8.7%	2.5%
BYSTANDER PARAMETERS						
Sigma / Pspon	1.8	7.9	5.2	6	8	1.9
q (per hit)	1.0	1.0	1.0	1.0	1.0	1.0
k (per hit)	1.9	0.72	1.9	1.9	1.9	1.9
Zeta	1.0	1.0	1.0	1.0	1.0	1.0
Nu (per hit)	1.3	0.1	0	0	0.5	4.7
Beta (per hit2)	-0.05	0.15	0.37	0.24	0.4	0
DirectDamageNormalHits - V	N/A	1.5	2	1.8	1.3	1.1
Width Half Maximum - Hits		0.4	0.6	0.6	0.4	0.3

3.1.b The Alpha Exposures of Zhou et al (2001) and Hei et al (1999) for A_L Cells

Two separate experiments used human-hamster hybrid A_L (CHO K1) cells to study mutagenesis from alpha particle irradiations. Hei et al (1999) used the Columbia University microbeam facility to irradiate the A_L cells with 1, 2, 4 and 8 exact numbers of 5.5 MeV alpha particles. These data, as were the Miller et al (1999) data in Figures 5B and 5C, of course would not reflect Bystander behavior. Later, Zhou et al (2001) used the microbeam facility to inject lower percentages of alpha particles to the *in vitro* A_L cells, i.e. 5, 10, 20 and 100%. The combined dose response results are given in Figures 5D through 5F. With these three graphs, we present the data with both Alpha Absorbed Dose and Exact Number of Nucleus Traversals for the full range of data (Figure 5D), for the low dose Bystander region (Figure 5E) and the full range on log scale (Figure 5F). We obtained a good fit to the low region using the empirically modified BaD Model best fit parameters for σ, ξ, γ, and k given in Table 1. Again, as with the Miller et al (1999) data, we had to use an empirical function to describe the behavior for the threshold of the direct damage region. These fit parameter values are also given in Table 1.

3.1.c Mutation Frequency for Alpha Particle Exposure of Wild-Type CHO Cells (Nagasawa and Little 1999, 2003)

Nagasawa and Little (1999, 2003) performed broadbeam alpha particle exposures of wild-type CHO cells and their repair deficient mutant xxr-5 cells, measuring mutation frequencies, in the Bystander dose range using 3.7 MeV alpha particles from a ^{238}Pu source in a special irradiator (Metting et al 1995). They also measured the frequency of chromosome aberrations with the same source and cell species (Nagasawa and Little 2002), which will be examined in Figure 6 herein. We did not analyze the mutation xxr-5 data because their data only covered the Bystander dose region. As Figures 5G through 5I, we provide the analysis of the mutation wild-type CHO data which extends to 120 cGy, well within the direct damage region for the 3.7 MeV alpha particles. Again we obtained a good least squares fit of the modified broadbeam BaD Model parameters to the low region Bystander data region. The best fit values for σ, ξ, γ, and k are given in Table 1. The same effect, suggestive of a threshold, was again observed for the initial direct damage region from 1 to 3 alpha particle traversals where a transition occurs into the direct damage linear-quadratic dose response behavior region. This is compatible with the threshold effect suggested by Miller et al (1999) but there is presently no experimental verification of this. The values for the threshold transition function and linear-quadratic α and β parameters are given in Table 1.

3.1.d Alpha Particle Induced Chromosome Aberrations for Wild-Type CHO and Repair Deficient xxr-5 Cells (Nagasawa and Little 2002)

The Nagasawa and Little (2002) measurements of chromosome aberrations in the same wild-type CHO cells provides a direct comparison to the mutation frequency data, in Section 3.1.c above, relative to Bystander and direct damage sensitivities.

Figure 6, The modified BaD Model best fit to the Nagasawa and Little (2002)

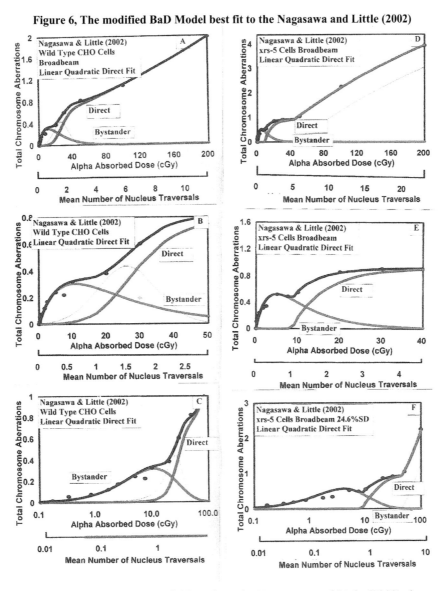

Figure 6 - The modified BaD Model best fit to the Nagasawa and Little (2002) chromosome aberration data for exposure of wild-type CHO and repair deficient xxr-5 cells to 3.7 MeV alphas. Experiments are described in Section 3.1.d and best fit parameters are given in Table 1.

Figures 6A through 6C provide the full range, low dose range and log scale presentation of the CHO data and the least squares fit, as was done above for the other alpha response data in Figure 5. The best fit parameter values are given in Table 1. As Figures 6D through 6F, we provide the similar data and best fits to the xxr-5 data of Nagasawa and Little (2002), the parameters given in Table 1. For the CHO and xxr-5 cells, we again see the model suggestion of a distinct transition between the Bystander damage to the direct damage with a threshold transition between about 1 and 3 alpha particle specific energy hits to the nucleus.

29

3.1.e The Relative Biological Effectiveness (RBE) of Alpha Particles

Martin et al (1995) and Miller et al (1995), using two positive ion accelerator facilities i.e. the Radiological Research Accelerator at Columbia University and the Tandem Van de Graaff Accelerator at Brookhaven National Laboratories, performed extensive measurements of oncogenic transformation frequencies for SHE Syrian hamster embryo (Martin et al 1995) and C3H 10T1/2 (Miller et al 1999) cells for a large range of ion LETs using ^{2}H, ^{3}He, ^{4}He and ^{19}F ions. We have chosen to examine the LET data of Miller et al (1999) for LET values of 3.8, 75, 90, 120, 150, 200 and 600 keV/μm. We have chosen these because their data sets provide for the alpha dose response in the low dose range where Bystander Effect would be present and also the higher dose range where the Direct Damage would be present. Both Martin et al (1995) and Miller et al (1999) analyzed the data by comparing the alpha dose response of the cells to low LET X-rays [300 kVp for Martin et al (1995) and 250 kVp for Miller et al (1999)] to assess the relative biological effectiveness of the alpha particles at the different high LETs of the ions including alpha particles (^{4}He ions). Their accelerator measurement of oncogenic transformation were over a range of ion particle doses ranging from 0.1 to 6.0 Gy. The RBE values, as presented in their Figure 3, were assessed by linearly graphing their dose response data and computing the slopes compared to the X-rays slope in their Figure 2. For alpha particles, the LET decreases mono-tonically with increasing alpha particle energy.

Figure 7, Alpha particle energies, LETs and a function of alpha RBE

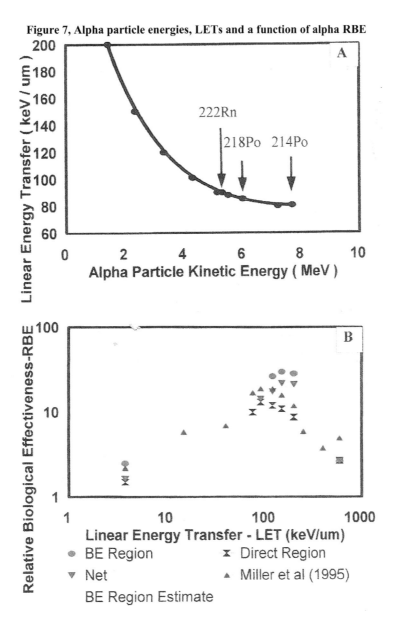

Figure 7 - Alpha particle energies, LETs and a function of alpha RBE. Panel A – The variation in LET as particle kinetic energy. Shown are the value for 222Rn, 218Po and 214Po radon and progeny alphas. Panel B – In analyzing the Miller et al (1995) 10T1/2 cell dose response data for a range of LETs, it is found due to the two distinct dose response regions i.e. Bystander and Direct Damage Regions, there are hence two distinct RBE values for the alpha particles relative to low LET radiation (see Figure 8 for two averages marked in red and green). Shown are the average RBEs in the BE Region and the Direct Damage Region along with Miller et al (1995) net RBE values. The data is discussed in Sections 3.1.e and 4.1.c.

Figure 7A provides the LET in keV/μm for alpha particles as a function of alpha kinetic energy in MeV. We show the alpha particles for ^{222}Rn and the progeny ^{218}Po and ^{214}Po.

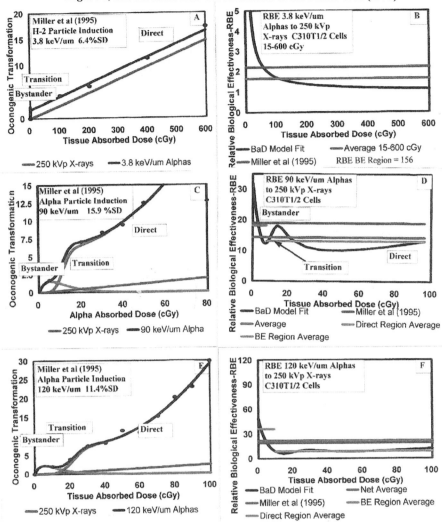

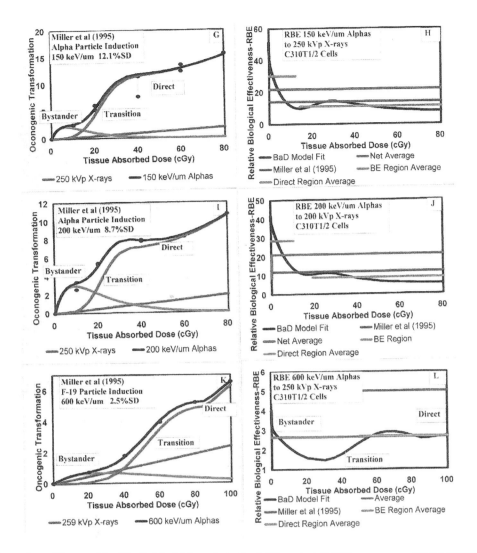

Figure 8 - The modified BaD Model best fit to the Miller et al (1995) exposure of C3H 10T1/2 cells to alpha particles of indicated range of LETs. Experiments are described in Section 3.1.e and 4.1.c and best fit parameters are given in Table 1.

Figure 8 panels A, C, E, G, I and K provides the fits of the Equation (4) modified BaD Model to the Miller et al (1999) data in terms of charged particle specific energy hits per nucleus (which is linear with dose). Due to the two separate response components experienced by the cells i.e. Bystander and direct damage as provided in the empirically modified BaD Model, the fits are not at all amenable to a constant slope linear fit   These region averaged RBE values are given in Figure 7B i.e. the average RBE values averaged separately over the Bystander Effect Damage Region and the Direct Damage Region, along with the RBE values reported by Miller et al (1995) in their Figure 3. We show a significant difference between the Bystander and Direct Damage values and between these and the Miller et al (1995) values. In Figure 8, panels B, D, F, H, J and L, we

33

provide the RBEs as a function of Tissue Absorbed Dose. In these Figure 8 RBE panels, we show in red the RBE average over the Bystander Damage Region and in green the average over the Direct Damage Region. Further analysis will be presented in Sectio 4.1.a.3. The best fit values of the empirically modified BaD Model parameters are given in Table 1.

3.1.f Summary of Alpha Particle Dose Response Studies and a Representative Alpha Particle Dose Response Shape

Figure 9, Summary of the alpha particle dose response data examined with the modified BaD Model

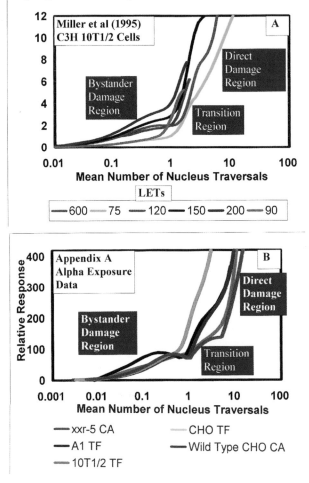

Figure 9 - Summary of the alpha particle dose response data examined in the Results Section. Panel A – The dose responses from Miller et al (1995) for different alpha and other charged particles at different LETs as given in the legend. Shown is a consistent Bystander Damage Region, a Threshold and Transition Region and a Direct Damage Region. The modified BaD Model parameters are given in Table 1. The magnitude of the Bystander Damage Region is shown to vary with LET similar to RBE. Panel B – The alpha particle dose response for four cell species and for transformation frequency and chromosome aberration production. A consistency is again shown when analyzed with respect to alpha particle Specific Energy Hits per cell Nucleus.

34

To examine the comparison between the data sets in Figure 9A we provide the modified broadbeam BaD Model best fits to the data of Miller et al (1995) obtained in all of their LET studies with the Mean Number of Nucleus Traversals as the abscissa scale . As Figure 9B with the same abscissa scale, we present the alpha particle modified broadbeam BaD Model best fits to the wild type CHO TF data of Nagasawa and Little (1999, 2003), the CHO and xxr-5 cell chromosome aberration data of Nagasawa and Little (2002) and the C3H 10T1/2 cell data of Miller et al (1999). In all of these, the best fit was by using a Normal Distribution accumulation function in the transition region between the Bystander Damage Region and the Direct Damage Region of dose response. The average of the mean values, in Table 1, for the transition is 1.68 alpha particle traversals with a transition width of 0.62 hits for the Normal distribution. From these consistent data in terms of alpha particle mean number of nucleus traversals for a number of different cell species and alpha LETs, we conclude that the dose response of alpha particles is relatively independent of cell species and the dose delivered per specific energy hit is principally dependent on the frequency of the hits, with there being two endogenic effects from the exogenic alphas i.e. a Bystander Damage effect below one alpha particle traversal and the Direct Damage effect above about two alpha traversals. We also show in Figure 9B the A_L transformation frequency (TF) data of Zhou et al (2001) and Hei et al (1999), which shows for exact numbers of traversals, a similar, consistant behavior. We can therefore premise that the incidence of carcinogenic producing neoplastic transformations and chromosome aberrations within human lung tissue must follow the same micro-dosimetric dose response with alpha particle traversals through the nucleus of the sensitive human lung cells. This consistency of alpha particle traversal tissue response shown in Figure 9 connotates a similarity found in the consistency of Poisson distributed single low LET traversals to activate the Adaptive Response radio-protection.

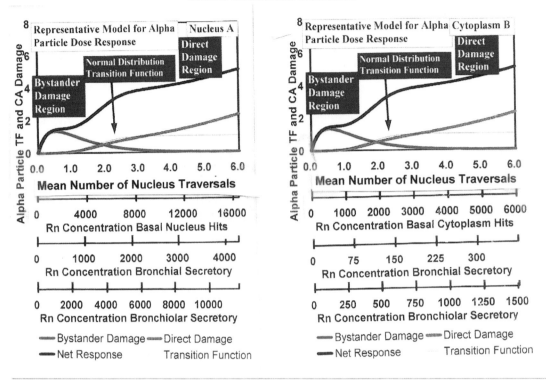

Figure 10 - A Representative Alpha Particle Dose Response for production of neoplastic transformation and induced chromosome aberrations based on the Table 1 averaged parameters for alpha particles with LET values near those for radon progeny alpha LETs shown in Figure 7. Also shown are abscissa scales for conversion to radon concentration (in Bq m-3) for hits to the nucleus and cytoplasm, based on James et al (2004) values, for the three lung cells sensitive to lung cancer induction. Panel A - Nucleus hits. Panel B – Cytoplasm hits.

With this premise, as Figure 10, we provide a consistent representative shape for alpha particle dose response as a function of Mean Number of Nucleus Traversals. In the low radon domestic dose region, the response will be concave from the Bystander Effect and linear with a moderate quadratic component in the high radon underground miners exposure region for the Direct Damage hits.

Since there are two distinctly shaped dose response regions, there are two distinct region averaged RBEs for the alpha particles relative to low LET radiations as seen in the Figure 8 panels and Figure 7B. In actuality, there are a continuous distribution of RBEs as the alpha dose response varies non-linearly and the low LET response varies approximately linearly. In the LET region for radon and progeny alpha particles (70 to 100 kev/μm) the difference is seen to range from about a factor of 1.7 to 3.2.

4. ANALYSIS

4.1. Summary of the Emperically Modified BaD Model Fit to Alpha Particle Dose Response Data, a Threshold and a Two Region Shape

4.1.a A Multiple Hit Threshold for Alpha Particle Activation of Direct Damage in Cells

In our analysis of published data of alpha particle induction of neoplastic transformation and chromosome aberrations, it was necessary to modify the basic Bystander broadbeam BaD Model, which we presented as Equation (2) above, to accommodate the observed dose response data for the broadbeam experiments. The basic problem was that a single alpha particle traversal through the cell does not initiate the Direct Damage dose response that should be expected since an alpha traversal deposits a relatively large amount of energy to the cell. The data of Miller et al (1999) in Figure 5C shows that a single alpha particle traversal does not initiate noticeable cell transformations and does not show a linear dose response for the first several alpha traversals per cell, as has been found to be true for alpha particle cell survival data. Past research has not as yet explained this behavior and this work also fails to do so. Our modification to the BaD Model was accomplished in the transition region with the use of the Normal Distribution accumulation function in Equation (11) below. All the alpha particle data examined in the Results Section show a distinct alpha particle threshold for initiation of the Direct Damage, between one to two alpha particle traversals. In the Figure 5 panels, we show Miller et al (1999) both the broadbeam and single alpha microbeam data. We above noted that the microbeam single alpha particle exposure is shown to have minimal cellular damage effect. This was noted by Miller et al (1999). We have tried introducing an alpha particle Poisson accumulation threshold transition function, as was done for the Direct Damage component of the composite AR and BE Microdose Model. We found that for various mean values from 1 to 3 Poisson distributed alpha particle mean specific energy hits that the fit was very unsatisfactory.

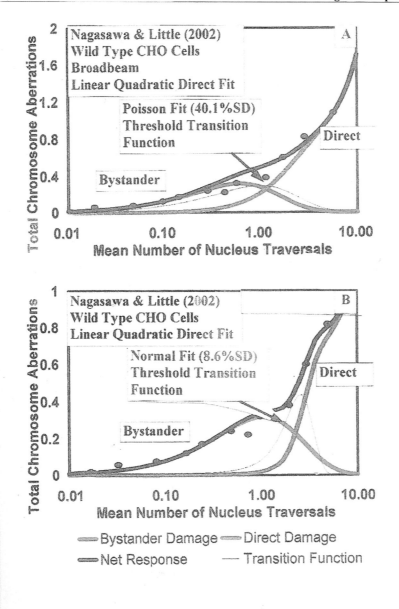

Figure 11 - A threshold and transition function for induction of Direct Damage from alpha particles. It is found in the fit of the bystander BaD Model that a mean of single alpha particle traversals do not activate the Direct Damage component. Panel A - A Poisson accumulation transition function tried with minimal success. Panel B – A normal distribution accumulation function provides a good fit in modeling the threshold transition from the Bystander Damage Region and the Direct Damage Region.

Figure 11A shows the fit for a Poisson distributed threshold mean of two alpha particle traversals to ± 40.1%SD for the Nagasawa and Little (2002) CHO data. The fit for a threshold of 1 alpha traversal was worse, the problem being that the Poisson function is too broad a function about the mean values. We next tried a Normal Distribution accumulation function, N(M,V,SD), with the property of a mean value, V, and a standard deviation (width at ½ maximum - SD) – again M is the mean hit as a function of alpha dose i.e. $M = D / <z_1>$. This Normal Distribution accumulation function, like the Poisson accumulation function, varies from 0 to unity as M (hits) increases. We found that the best fit value of the mean number of alpha particles to model the threshold was 1.68 hits with a SD of 0.62 hits (this being the average values of V and SD in Table 1). Figure 11B provides the best fit for the Nagasawa and Little (2002) data to ± 8.6%SD using the Normal distribution function for the threshold. For the analysis of all the alpha particle broadbeam dose response data reported here, from Equation (2) we have used an emperically modified broadbeam BaD Model given by

$$TF = \gamma \, q \, N(M,V,SD) \, M + \sigma \, [\, 1 - Exp \, (-k \, M) \,] \, Exp \, (-q \, M) \qquad (7)$$

using $M = <N>$ and with the normal distribution function $N(M,V,SD)$ in the modified broadbeam BaD Model Direct Damage component and the other parameters defined above and in Appendix B. We do not offer an empirical or analytical explanation for the need of this modification nor did Miller et al (1999) for their observations. One thought is that Bystander cell killing could eliminate spontaneous transformants and lead to a reduction in the overall transformation frequency after low fluences of alpha particles and the response becomes linear at the higher fluences.

4.1.b Use of the Broadbeam BaD Model Equation for Analysis of Experimental Alpha Dose Response Measurements

The broadbeam BaD Model Equation (2) is derived by Brenner et al (2001) from the microbeam Equation (1) using standard microdosimetric principals, taking into account the microdosimetric fluctuations conditional on a given absorbed dose. This involves averaging over a Poisson distribution of hits for a fixed absorbed dose level. We have here used the mean specific energy deposition constant for nucleus traversals, $<z_1>$ (units cGy per hit), to estimate the mean number of alpha particle nucleus traversals to the cell nuclei by division of the tissue absorbed dose (units of cGy) by $<z_1>$. This provides the independent variable Mean Number of Nucleus Traversals used in our analysis. We have essentially averaged away the microdosimetric fluctuations and any impact on biological responses before their use of their empirical model in Equations (2) and (3). Others (Little and Wakeford 2001, Little 2004, Brenner and Sachs 2002, 2003, Brenner et at 2001) have estimated the size of the cell nuclei and alpha LET values to estimate $<z_1>$ in using the broadbeam Equation (1) in examining Bystander Effect although technically not microdosimetrically correct either.

The BaD Model and our subsequent non-conventional modifications here have acquired the empirically derived functions in our Equation (7). Neither the model and our Equation (7) consider the fact that the types of chromosome aberrations and mutations produced by the Bystander cells are different from those produced by the direct radiation damage. Direct damage produces chromosome type of aberrations and deletion type mutations while Bystander damage produces chromatid type aberrations This suggests that the Bystander damage may also be protective by the protective apoptosis and cell death to eliminate transformed cells such as spontaneous transformants. As noted, this may explain the low microbeam dose response observed by Miller et al (1999) and, at least empirically, the need for two hits to activate the Direct Damage component of our broadbeam data fits. The Equation (7) functions have thus been successfully used to capture the complexity of the dose-response experimental data examined here and as discussed in the following section 4.1.c, obtain a Representative bAlpha Particle Dose Response behavior in terms of Bystander and direct damage.

4.1.c A Representative Microdose Alpha Particle Dose Response Relative to Increasing Alpha Charged Particle Traversals in the Absence of Adaptive Response

In our extensive study of Adaptive Response dose response behavior with the Microdose Model, it was found for over 25 cell species dose response data sets, that certain properties of the response were invariant. In simple words, the AR dose response had a representative behavior. One was that the threshold and protective state occurred at the dose value of $<z_1>$ (thus single hit "triggering") by Poisson accumulation of the hits. The other was that the Adaptive Response protection effect became diminished at about 10 cGy of low LET priming dose where the deleterious Direct Damage began to dominate. These properties are shown in Figures 17 and 21 and discussed in Section 2.2.e of Chapter 3 - Part II. For the Bystander Effect Figure 9 shows similarities in dose response shape properties for alpha particle dose response suggesting an invariance given by Figure 10.

Similarly, there have been speculation about the eventual overall shape of the dose response curve for ionizing radiation by Morgan(2006) and Brenner and Sachs (2003, 2006) with the new Bystander and Adaptive Response data.

Figure 12, The human lung cancer risk response curves

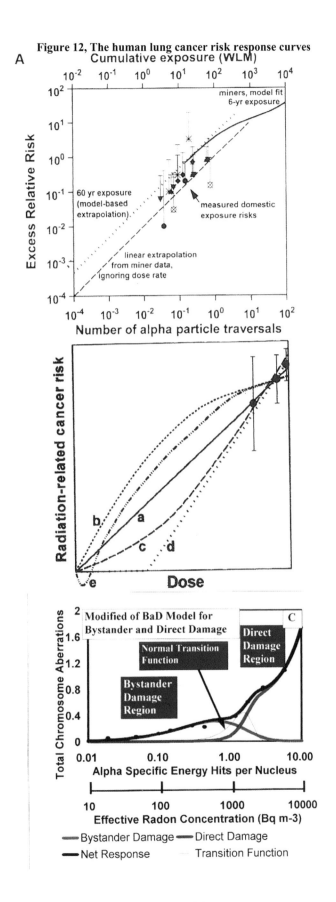

41

Figure 12 - The human lung cancer risk response curves. Panel A – The suggested Excess Relative Risk for human lung cancer from radon as suggested by Brenner and Sachs (2002). Panel B – Possible shapes of the lung cancer radiation risks based on non-linear premises from bystander, Adaptive Response and other cellular mechanism effects (Brenner et al 2003). – Both reproduced with permission. Panel C – The modified BaD Model dose response from alpha particles as determined from microbeam exposures

Figure 12A is a reproduction of Figure 4A from Brenner and Sachs (2002) for Excess Relative Risk where generally a linear cancer risk is shown. The non-linear curvature at the high radon levels is from the presumed high radon "inverse" dose rate effect (IDRE) affecting the underground miners. In a later paper, considering the prospects that hormesis type protective behavior (curve e) may occur in some instances and the potential for deleterious Bystander Effect (curve b), the Figure 12B provides a dose response graph reproduced from Figure 3 of Brenner and Sachs (2003). These possibilities are in concert with the alternatives presented by Morgan (2006) relative to the ultimate roles of the Bystander Effect and Adaptive Response radio-protection. Since human exposures to radon are broadbeam exposures, from our Results Section evaluation with the modified Bystander broadbeam BaD Model, we can estimate a possible invariant, representative relative risk dose response by the simple assumption that alpha particle induction of human lung cancer should behave similar to the production of neoplastic transformation and chromosome aberration shown for a number of cell species for alpha particles in panels in Figures 5, 6 and 8. As Figure 12C, we have shown the emperically modified broadbeam BaD Model fit curves for the six data sets of Miller et al (1995) in their LET and RBE study from Figure 8. In Figure 9B, we have shown the emperically modified broadbeam BaD Model fit curves for the data sets in Figure 5 and 6 panels for the different cell species studied. Both Figure 9A and 9B show the broadbeam curves plotted in terms of Mean Number of Nucleus Traversals. The broadbeam curves in Figure 9B for different cell species and two biological "endpoints" are very similar, with the deviations most likely from experimental variances. The broadbeam curves in Figure 9A appear to only vary in a systematic way with LET. The LETs of the exposures are given in Table 1 and in the legend of Figure 9A for the Miller et al (1995) data. The LETs of the radon and progeny alphas are approximately 90 keV/μm. In Part I of Table 1, we see that the LET of the Nagasawa and Little (1999, 2002) experiments is 112 keV/μm. We have computed the average and variances of the Bystander Damage and Direct Damage parameters given for the three Nagasawa and Little (1999, 2002) sets in Part I and the 90 and 120 keV/μm sets of Miller et al (1995) in Part II of Table 1. Figure

42

10 provides a resulting Representative Alpha Particle Dose Response based on these analysis of the broadbeam dose response data.. We use the average empirically modified broadbeam BaD Model parameter values for Equation (6) i.e. $\sigma = 2.8$, $q = 1.00$ per hit, $k = 1.9$ per hit, $\xi = 1.00$, Nu $(\alpha) = 0.10$, $\beta = 0.144$, $V = 1.68$ hits and SD $= 0.62$ hits obtained from Table 1. We show that, since residential radon levels would induce damage primarily in the Bystander Damage Region to the lung, the dose response curve should be expected to have a downward concave curvature as shown in Figure 10 - similar to curve b of Brenner and Sachs (2003) and our Figure 12C. The BEIR VI (1999) Figure 3-2 and the dose response curves of the case-control studies in Figure 2 herein fail to, of course, reflect this concavity due to the LNT assumption. In Part III, we show that the case-control data provides a best fit to a downward concave curvature.

With this premise of a Representative Alpha Particle Dose Response curve with respect to alpha particle traversals per nucleus as the independent variable parameter, we use a concave response curve as a starting point in the residential radon level region (Bystander Damage Region) and estimate a more realistic general dose response curve than in Figures 12A and 12B. We can hypothesize that the alpha particle dose response of the lung cells for lung cancer risk must have the overall shape similar to the Figure 10, with respect to alpha particle traversals per nucleus. Then, with this representative shape, the Figure 10 curve needs to be normalized to the spontaneous risk of lung cancer in consideration of the relative shape values of Figure 10. Since these will be important in evaluating, in Part III (Leonard et al 2010b), the radon lung cancer risk data from the case-control studies shown in Figures 2A and 2B, we provide in the abscissa in Figure 10, separate scales for the effective radon concentrations for alpha particle hits to the potential lung "target" cells i.e. basal, bronchial secretory and bronchiolar secretory cells and for the nucleus and entire cell (nucleus and cytoplasm. Panels A and B). These are based on the traversals to radon concentration conversions provided by James et al (2004). We thus have obtained a Repersentative Alpha Particle Dose Response shape, without the presence of any low LET radiations to activate Adaptive Response protective effects that may influence the overall human lung cancer risk curve (which will be examined in Part II). We will see that we also must consider the high radon IDRE effect at the high radon levels in developing a relative risk curve encompassing the high alpha dose data in the Appendix A when applied to the underground miners. But the IDRE occurs above normal domestic and workplace radon levels for humans.

4.1.d A Significantly Variable RBE for Alpha Particles with Dose and Alpha Traversals, Especially for the Low Residential Radon Levels

We further examine the results of the analysis with respect to LET. For the Miller et al (1995) RBE data, it is found in Section 3.1.e of the Results Section that although the shapes are the same, as noted above, the relative magnitudes of the Bystander Damage and the Direct Damage components varies with LET of the high LET radiation. In Figure 8, we show, on the left as Panels A, C, E, G, I and K, the Microdose Model best fit to the Miller et al (1995) LET and RBE study. In these left panels, we provide the 250 kVp X-ray response that Miller et al (1995) used to compute the RBEs. Side-by-side for ready reference, the right panels provide the computed RBEs as a function of alpha particle Tissue Absorbed Dose, as the solid black curve, the simple ratio of alpha dose response to X-ray dose response (the ratio of the two dose response curves). It is clear that there is no reasonably constant effective RBE for the entire range of doses as was estimated and reported by Miller et al (1995). We have computed the averages over the two separate Bystander and Direct Damage Regions using the single alpha traversal Direct Damage threshold as the boundary, These are shown in solid red and green on the graphs. As Figure 8F, we see that the RBE varies from about 35 to about 10 for 90 keV/μm LET alpha particles. Figure 7A shows the variation of LET with alpha particle kinetic energy. Figure 7B shows, for all the Miller et al (1995) LET data sets, the magnitudes of the average RBEs for the Bystander Damage and Direct Damage Regions (from Figure 8) for the Miller et al (1995) LETs showing the large variation. The LETs of the three radon alpha particles for 5.49 MeV ^{222}Rn, 6.00 MeV ^{218}Po and 7.69 MeV ^{214}Po are 88, 85.2 and 80.5 keV/μm, respectively. For the radon progeny alpha particles, the RBE is very large at very low radon concentrations and decreases by a factor of about 3.5 at higher radon levels, so cannot reasonably be represented by a single RBE value as Miller et al (1995) reported.

4.1.e The Best Fit Modified Broadbeam BaD Model Parameters for the Alpha Dose Response Data

Using the emperically modified broadbeam BaD Model, Equation (7), to analyze the alpha particle dose response data presented in the Results Section, we have provided the best fit parameters given in Table 1. Given are the best fit least squares standard deviations. It is found that the modified broadbeam BaD Model provides an excellent analytical tool in describing the dose response of the four cell species (CHO,

C3H 10T1/2, A_L and xxr-5) dose response to alpha radiation and adequately depicts the Bystander Effect broadbeam bio-physical behavior.

4.2 Correlation Between Alpha Particle Traversals Through Lung Tissue and Indoor Radon Concentration

4.2.a Traversals of Alpha Particles and Specifically Radon Alpha Particle Exposure to Human Lung Tissue

Since the issuance of BEIR VI (1999), James et al (2004), as noted above, has provided a new assessment of the effect of radon alpha particle traversals (hits) through human lung tissue with some changes in the effects as a function of radon concentrations (in kBq m^{-3} units) for residential and underground miners exposures. This re-assessment thus supplements the International Commission on Radiological Protection (ICRP) Report 66, Human Respiratory Tract Model for Radiological Protection (ICRP 1994). They provide, in tabular form, the probabilities of single and multiple alpha particle hits, as a function of radon concentration, for the three most sensitive human lung cells i.e. bronchial basal, bronchial secretory and bronchiolar secretory cells. It is generally accepted (BEIR VI 1999, James et al 2004) that lung epithelial cells are responsive to potentially carcinogenic damage over the 30 day mitotic cycle. Figure 4A and 4B provide graphs of the probabilities of single alpha particle hits to the cell nucleus and to the cytoplasm (entire cell) during a 30 day exposure for the three cell species. It is the consensus that the sensitive region of the cell, with respect to radiation induced chromosome damage, is the cell nucleus, so we have used the nucleus in our evaluations as we have done in the past for Adaptive Response radio-protection studies.

The James et al (2004) re-analysis of alpha particle lung cell traversals allows us to correlate the alpha particle dose response data studied in the Results Section and the representative alpha particle traversal response shape in Figure 10 to human radon exposure concentrations. From the James et al (2004) hit rate values, we provide the correlation between radon concentrations to inflict the alpha particle Specific Energy hits for the representative shape model in Figure 10 with radon concentration abscissa scales for the three cell species. We are interested in estimating the number of specific energy hits that human lung cells receive in the residential radon setting and that the underground miners receive in their mine workspace setting, based on US radon surveys.

Figure 13, Distribution of radon concentrations in US homes

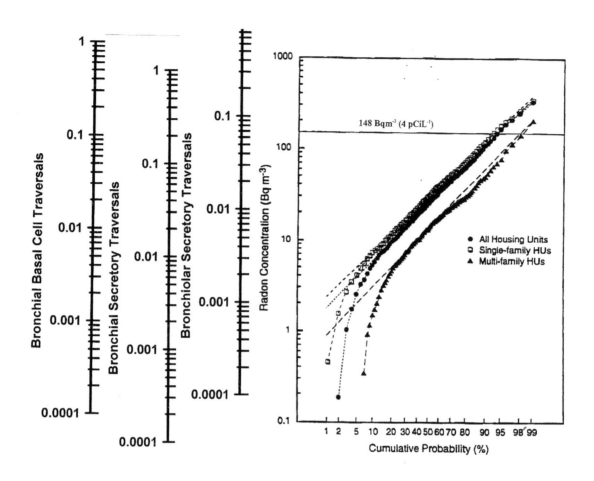

Figure 13- Reproduction of the BEIR VI Figure 1-4 distribution of radon concentrations in US homes. Added are scales of alpha particle traversals to the three radon sensitive human lung cells from James et al (2004). This shows that during the 30 day cycle only fractions of hits occur per cell and human lung cancer risks are from Bystander Damage effects. Reproduced with permission.

Figure 13 provides a reproduction of Figure 1-4 of BEIR VI (1999) showing the distribution of radon concentrations in US homes, but with added ordinate axis scales for alpha particle traversals to the three lung cell species. We see that only fractions of traversals occur to the lung cells at radon levels experienced in US homes during the 30 day cell cycles. We can compare this with the cellular alpha particle traversals of bthe underground miners. Various studies have reported radon concentration distributions in the underground miners workspaces. In earlier work, as Figure 13A of Leonard (2007c), we have tabulated the underground miners radon concentration distribution from reports of underground miners workspace measurements conducted by Andria George and his group at the US Environmental Measurements Laboratory.

Figure 14, Based on underground miners exposures presented in Figure 13A of Leonard (2007c)

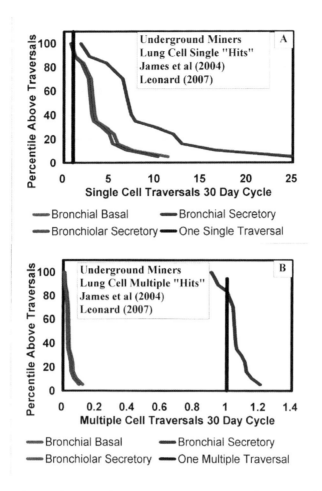

Figure 14 - Based on underground miners exposures presented in Figure 13A of Leonard (2007c), We show Panel A – The percentile of mine workstations where one lung cell alpha particle traversal will occur in the 30 day cycle. Panel B – Percentile of workstations where multiple traversals will occur. Thus for the underground miners their lung cancer risks are from Direct Damage alpha particle traversals not from Bystander Damage.

Figure 14A herein provides graphs of the percentile of miners workstations with cell traversals above the abscissa Single Cell Traversal for a 30 Day Cycle for the three lung cell species. As Figure 14B, we show the Percentiles for Multiple Cell Traversals. The vertical solid black line is for 1 traversal in the 30 day period. We see for single traversals that at least 95% of all miners workstations would result in at least one cell traversal per cell cycle. About 50% would receive at least 3 traversals to the bronchial basal and bronchiolar secretory cells and at least 50% of the bronchial secretory cells would receive 7 cell traversals. Thus, humans exposed to radon in the residential setting will receive lung cell alpha particle damage via the Bystander Effect and underground miners will receive lung cell alpha particle damage via direct alpha particle traversals -

Direct Damage Effect. For the miners, multiple alpha particle traversals are experienced in inducing the observed high lung cancer incidence.

4.2.b The Representative Alpha Particle Dose Response in Assessing Human Lung Cancer Risks from Residential Level and Underground Miners Radon Concentrations – Excluding Adaptive Response Radio-protection Effects

The BEIR VI (1999) Committee has summarized their assessment of human lung cancer risks as a function of radon concentration in their Figure 3-2 of BEIR VI (1999) shown here as Figure 1C. The Relative Risks are estimated to have a slope of about 0.20 per 100 Bq m^{-3} of indoor radon. For the underground miners data alone, they provide a slightly lower Relative Risk of about 0.18 per 100 Bq m^{-3}.

Figure 15, Reproduction of BEIR VI Relative Risk Figure 3-2 showing traversal data for the lung cell

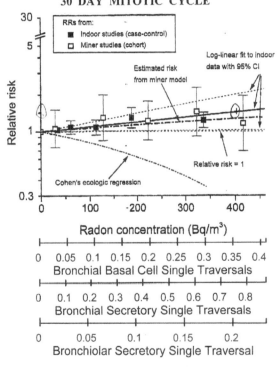

Figure 15 - Reproduction of BEIR VI Relative Risk Figure 3-2. Added are the James et al (2004) traversal data for the lung cell nucleus as target as abscissa scales, showing that humans at domestic radon levels receive fractions of traversal per cell per cycle.

Figure 15 reproduces their Figure 3-2 with also the lung cell traversals based on the James et al (2004) data. This again shows that the cellular damage induced by the alpha particles from radon at residential levels must be almost solely from alpha particle Bystander damage from fractions of traversals per cell, since such a small fraction are directly hit. Based on the large amount of dose response data examined in the Results Section relative to cellular sensitivity to the Bystander Effect, we can estimate a more realistic Relative Risk curve than given by the BEIR VI (1999) Figure 3-2. If we assume that the indoor case-control studies and the low exposure underground miners data in the radon concentration around 400 Bq m^{-3} are reasonably accurate, we can provide an improvement over previous premises such as shown in Figure 10.

James et al (2004) has stated that presently the relative lung cancer carcinogenesis for the three lung cell species is not known and recommends use of an average. We have converted the adjusted representative alpha particle traversal data in Figure 10 to Radon Exposure Concentration. In Figure 10, we, as separate abscissa scales, provide the equivalent radon concentrations separately for the three cells using James et al (2004) Table 12 values of 0.00036, 0.0014 and 0.00051 single traversals per Bq m^{-3} of radon per 30 day cell mitotic cycles. We show scales for nucleus and total (cytoplasm) traversals.

4.2.c *Normalization of the Representative Radon Alpha Particle Dose Response to Radon Relative Lung Cancer Risks*

We wish to offer a more realistic general dose response curve for lung tissue exposure to radon progeny alpha particles than the options in Figures 12A and 12B. As noted above, without a more accurate re-assessment of human lung cancer Relative Risk data since BEIR VI (1999), in applying the representative shape curve in Figure 10 to radon exposures, a conservative approach is to normalize the Figure 10 curve to the BEIR VI (1999) Figure 3-2 RR at the 400 Bq m^{-3} radon level since the higher values are believed to be more accurate.

Figure 16, A "standard" dose response model, based on the representative dose response

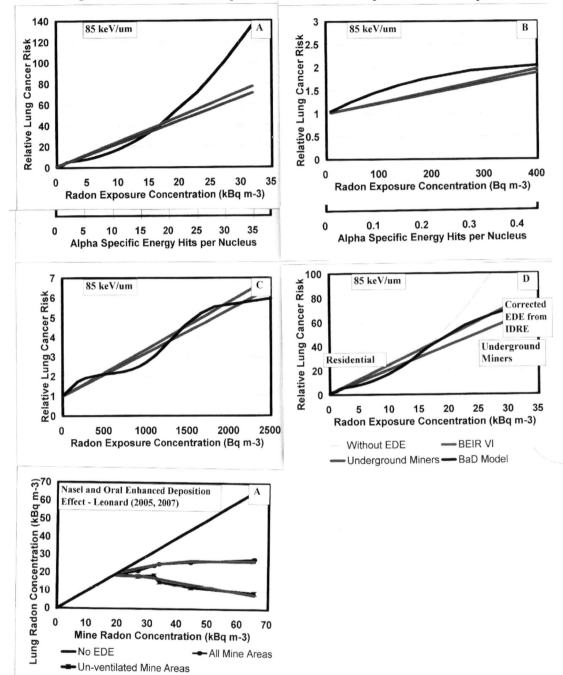

Figure 16 - A "standard" dose response model, based on the representative dose response in Figure 10, for alpha particle induction of lung cancer cellular damage to humans from radon based on Specific Energy Hits to the lung bronchial basal, bronchial secretory and bronchiolar secretory cells sensitivity given by James et al (2004). Panel A – the dose response over the entire range of alpha particle traversals from domestic to underground miner levels. Panel B – Normalization of the "standard" model to the BEIR VI Radon Lung Cancer Risk at 400 Bq M-3. Panel C – Presentation of the low and middle dose response region showing the Bystander Damage Region and the Transition Region into the Direct Damage Region. Panel D – The full dose response range showing the correction for the nasal and oral breathing passage Enhanced Deposition Effect (EDE) causing the radon "Inverse" Dose Rate Effect.

Panel E – The EDE correction at high radon levels. Reproduced from Leonard (2007c) with permission. Reproduced from Leonard (2008c) with permission.

As Figure 16A, we show the alpha particle dose response from Figure 10, up to high radon levels, for Radon Exposure Concentration and Alpha Specific Energy Hits per Nucleus, with also the BEIR VI (1999) residential estimate in red and the BEIR VI underground miners estimate in blue. [We must remember that the representative shape curve is for alpha particle production of chromosome aberrations and not directed applicable to human cancer risk. We will address that issue when the dose response data for radon case-control studies are examined in Part III of our study.] We show a very large difference in the high radon region in Figure 16A. As Figure 16B for low radon levels, we show the normalized curve, reflecting Bystander damage concave dose response in the residential range of human radon exposure. Figures 16C and 16D provide the response with an estimate of the high radon region accounting for reduction from the "inverse" dose rate effect as was done in Figure 12B. In Figure 16D, we show the dose response in the mid-range where the transition between Bystander Effect Damage and Direct Damage occurs and show also the high radon range relative to underground miners exposures. Section 4.2.d will consider the radon "inverse" dose rate effect (IDRE) and the Enhanced Deposition Effect (EDE) with respect to the high radon regions of Figures 16A, 16C and 16D.

4.2.d Consideration of the High Radon "Inverse" Dose Rate Effect

Lubin et al (1995), in evaluating underground miners lung cancer incidence rates, found that at high radon levels the lung cancer Relative Risk decreased at high radon concentrations, referred to as the "inverse" dose rate effect (IDRE). We show the Relative Risk reduction from IDRE as Figure 13D. In radon modeling, BEIR VI (1999) has included a correction factor for IDRE, as shown in Figure 16D, for this effect in their Relative Risk model. Only alpha particle dose saturation has been premised for the effect. In studying radon progeny depositions in a radon test chamber, Leonard (1996) observed an excessive surface deposition on the chamber walls at high radon levels. In subsequent measurements, it was found, consistent with the results of Porstendorfer (2001) that at high radon levels above about 20 kBq m^{-3} the airborne radon progeny disassociates from its aerosol attachment creating a highly mobile unattached progeny particulate. Using ICRP (1994) report 66, it was shown that the smaller diameter progeny experiences

51

enhanced deposition to the nasal and oral breathing passages, thus reducing the radon reaching the lung. This is referred to as the nasal and oral passage enhanced deposition effect (EDE). Figure 16E shows the Lung Radon Concentration relative to the air radon concentration within the mine for un-ventilated and all mine work areas. This IDRE effect will occur for the high alpha particle doses in the underground miners radon levels.

Using the alpha adjusted dose response data for Representative Alpha Particle Dose Response in Figure 10 and the EDE corrections in Figure 16E, we have corrected the high dose relative risk data, above 20 kBq m-3, for the EDE as shown in Figure 16D. We show the overall Relative Lung Cancer Risk for the residential levels and underground miners. This then we consider our best estimate of radon Relative Lung Cancer Risk, without the presence of AR protective low LET radiations, taking into account that residential level human lung exposures are from Bystander Damage and underground miners are from alpha particle Direct Damage including the "inverse" dose rate effect correction from the enhanced deposition effect influencing the underground miners exposure above about 20 kBq m^{-3} of radon.

4.2.e *Differences in Type Chromosome Damage Between Bystander and Direct Cellular Damage from Alpha Particle Ionizing Radiation*

Ward (1985, 1988, 1995) was one of the first investigators to examine the distinct types of chromosome damage produced by ionizing radiation. It is now known that there is a distinct difference in the damage products from Bystander signal damage and from direct alpha particle damage. Morgan (2003a, 2003b) has discussed various damage effects including genomic instability for Bystander and direct damage. The nature of the cellular communication that is involved in producing these Bystander responses is not known, there is strong evidence for chemical signaling processes, oxidative metabolism and gap-junction mediated cell-to-cell communication processes playing roles in the Bystander phenomenon. There is evidence that Bystander cell damage produces an enhanced frequency of chromatid-type aberrations compared to chromosome-type aberrations (Schmid and Roos 2008). Irradiated medium has been found to produce chromatid aberrations when transferred to hamster hybrid (AL) cells (Suzuki et al 2004). Jostes et al (1994) found a difference between Bystander and targeted induced mutations Huo et al (2001) found that cells damaged by the Bystander Effect from alpha particles resulted in primarily point mutations versus deletions at high alpha fluences suggesting their induction by different mechanisms. Schollinberger et al 2006) have modeled the induction on chromosome aberrations for direct and Bystander mechanisms. It is quite certain then that the carcinogenic potential of Bystander and direct alpha traversed chromosome damage must be different. Since the underground miners primarily receive direct traversed damage and humans exposed to domestic and workplace level radon receive primarily Bystander cellular damage, then the cancer risk most likely can not be directly compared on a chromosome aberration, mutation or transformation frequency basis. Thus the underground miners dose response data may not be useable for low level radon cancer risks in the radon concentration range presented in BEIR VI (1999) Figure 3-2 with these corrections which were not done in NRC (1991).

4.2.f Use of Brenner et al (2001) Emperically Modified Broadbeam BaD Model Equation (7) Herein

The Brenner et al (2001) BaD Model broadbeam equation [Equation (2) herein] was used in the work of Little and Wakeford (2001), Little (2004), Brenner and Sachs (2002, 2003), Brenner et al (2001) in examining the broadbeam data relative to underground miner and domestic level radon cancer risks. The primarily object here in this Part I analysis was to obtain a representative dose response shape applicable to potentially carcinogenic chromosome aberration, mutation and transformation frequency cellular damage in the radon concentration levels related to human domestic level radon exposure. Based on the analysis, we showed that the representative shape is relatively independent of cell species, for the cell species examined, and alpha particle LET in the range of the LETs of the radon progeny alpha particles. We used a non-conventional, empirically modified broadbeam BaD Model Equation (7) to perform this analysis. Most significant was the need for the use of a Normal Distribution transition function in the region where Bystander damage diminishes and the direct damage begin to dominate. The need for this is not known, Miller et al (1999) premised that perhaps two alpha traversals per cell are necessary to produce the Direct Damage. The real reason is not known. Other possibilities are a reduction in the spontaneous damage, the killing off of cells by apoptosis or some other unknown. The Normal Distribution transition function provided the proper dose response shape behavior in that region with a mean number of 1.68 hits and a transitrion region between one and two alpha particle hits.

From our work here, we show that the Bystander BaD Model of Brenner and sachs provides an excellent framework for analysis of Bystander dose response.

53

5. PART I SUMMARY

Since the publication of the BEIR VI (1999) report in 1999 on health risks from radon, a significant amount of new data has been published showing various mechanisms that may affect the ultimate assessment of radon as a carcinogen, at low domestic and workplace radon levels, in particular the potentially deleterious Bystander Effect (BE) and the potentially beneficial Adaptive Response radio-protection (AR). Although most of the BE research has been studying *in vitro* radiation dose responses using microbeam single alpha particle irradiations, it has been readily premised that human lung cancer is caused, at least partially, by BE damage to lung cells. Recent analysis of AR research results with a Microdose Model has shown that single low LET induced radiation charged particles traversals through the cell nucleus activates AR protection. In this three part study, we have conducted an analysis based on what is presently known and what new research is needed that can assist in the further evaluation human cancer risks from radon. Using a modified version of the Brenner et al (2001) Bystander broadbeam BaD Model merged into a composite BE and AR Microdose Model, published as a review article in Dose-Response Journal (Leonard 2008b), we here have analyzed the microbeam alpha particle data of Miller et al (1999) and Zhou et al (2001) and the broadbeam alpha particle data of others and show that, in terms of alpha particle traversals, the shape of the cellular response to alphas is relatively independent of cell species and LET of the alphas in the range of radon progeny alpha energies and primarily dependent on alpha particle traversals through the cell proper. The result is that the same broadbeam alpha particle traversal dose response should be true for human broadbeam lung tissue exposure to radon progeny alpha particles. Further it is found in the Bystander Damage Region of the alpha particle response that there is not a single alpha particle RBE but a variation as shown in Figure 8.

6. PART I CONCLUSIONS

Our findings here in Part I, for alpha particle Bystander Effect influence on human lung cancer risk, are as follows:

- A common alpha particle dose response for production of deleterious oncogenic neoplastic transformations and chromosome aberrations exists in terms of alpha particle charged particle traversals through the cells nucleus. The alpha particle hit response, basically independent of cell species and the small range of LETs for the radon and progeny alphas, consist of two distinct regions i.e. a Bystander Damage Region and a Direct Damage Region with a transition region between one and two alpha traversals.

- A Representative Alpha Particle Dose Response shape can be estimated encompassing the low, residential radon level Bystander Effect Region and the high, underground miner radon level Direct Damage Region.

- The radon progeny alpha particle cellular response of human lung tissue relative to the potential carcinogenic neoplastic transformation and chromosome aberrations is similar and then so should the human lung cancer risks from radon. The shape of the human lung cancer risk curves for case-control studies should be non-linear and similar to the Representative Alpha Particle Dose Response shape.

- It is most probable that the underground miners lung cancer risk data may not be applicable to low domestic level radon human lung cancer risks due to different cellular damage mechanisms.

Chapter 3 - PART II - INFLUENCE FROM COMBINED ADAPTIVE RESPONSE AND BYSTANDER EFFECT

1. INTRODUCTION

We present here Part II of this three part study of the potential effects of Adaptive Response radio-protection and Bystander Effect on the human health risks from radon. In Chapter 2 - Part I, we have primarily examined experimental *in vitro* data that show the effect of radon progeny and other high LET alpha particles on the induction of transformation frequencies and chromosome aberrations in a number of cell species thus illustrating the potential for alpha particle induction of carcinogens in human lung tissue. It is found that the cellular dose response from alpha particles is relatively independent of cell species and LET of the alpha radiation to within about ± 10% and is non-linear. Thus a Representative Alpha Particle Dose Response shape is obtained which should be applicable to the alpha particle dose response in human lung tissue. This Representative Alpha Particle Dose Response shape is shown in Figure 10. It is then normalized to the BEIR VI Figure 3-2 estimated lung cancer Relative Risk at 400 Bq m-3, believed to be reliable for both the case-control and underground miners lung risk data. The normalized dose response is presented as Figure 16 of Part I. In the Part I analysis, it is found that the Brenner et al (2001) BaD microdose Bystander Model is an excellent tool for the analysis of Bystander Effect in tissue with however the necessity to require two alpha particle hits to initiate the Direct Damage component of the dose response, consistent with observations of Miller et al (1999). It is also found that the human lung cancer relative risk should not be Linear No-Threshold and that underground miners risk data may not be valid for estimating risks at domestic and workplace radon levels.

Compatible, as premised by others (Little and Wakeford 2001, Little 2004, Brenner and Sachs 2002, 2003, Brenner 1994, Brenner et at 2001), that Bystander Effect Damage occurs in human lung tissue from the high LET radon alpha radiations, we here further premise in this Part II text, also based on an abundance of *in vitro* data, that Adaptive Response radio-protection most probably is activated in human lung cells by predominantly low LET radiations received on a continually basis by humans from natural background and man-made radiations.

2. MATERIALS AND METHODS

2.1 Models for Adaptive Response Dose Response Behavior and Combined Bystander and Adaptive Response Behavior

In the following sections we will provide a summary of the Adaptive Response Microdose Model (Leonard 2007a, 2007b) and a composite Adaptive Response and Bystander Microdose Model (Leonard 2008a, 2008b, 2008c). These will be used in the Appendix A and the Results sections to examine combined BE and AR effects relative to human lung cancer risks from radon.

2.1.a Adaptive Response Suppression of Cellular Damage

Since the Adaptive Response effect involves the micro-dosimetric induction of a radio-protective behavior in cells from the passage of small numbers of radiation induced charged particles through the cell, we have earlier developed the Adaptive Response Microdose Model (Leonard 2005, 2007a, 2007b). As Equation (1) below, we provide a modified form of the AR Microdose Model from Leonard (2007a):

$$\text{Dose Response} = DR = P_{spon} \{ [1 - P_{prot-s\infty} \, PAF_S \, (M,N)]$$
$$+ [1 - P_{prot-r\infty} \, PAF_R \, (M,Q)] \, f(M) \, PAF_D \, (M,U) \, (\alpha \, D + \beta \, D^2) \} \tag{1}$$

where P_{spon} is the zero dose natural spontaneous damage, $P_{prot-s\infty}$ and $P_{prot-r\infty}$ are the Adaptive Response protection fractions for the reduction of the spontaneous and radiation induced damage. Broad beam exposures are assumed to deliver Poisson distributed cellular events (Brenner et al. 2001, Miller et al. 1999, Little and Wakeford 2001). The f(M) is the AR dissipation function in the Direct Damage Region. PAF_S, PAF_R and PAF_D are the Poisson accumulation functions for the transition of the Adaptive Response spontaneous, the radiation damage protection and the deleterious direct damage, respectively, given by

$$PAF \, (M,n) = 1 - Exp \, (-M) \sum_{\gamma=0}^{n} M^{n-\gamma} / (n-\gamma)! = 1 - \sum_{j=0}^{n} P \, (M,j) \tag{2}$$

In this general form for the Poisson accumulation function, M is the mean number of events occurring (such as cell hits) from the radiation dose and n is the number of incidental events (hits) necessary to produce the effect (in our case cell radio-biology "endpoints"). It is important to note that M is the mean number of events for a statistically significant large cell population and is not an integer but a continuous function of dose. The linearity of M as a function of dose is given by $M = D / <z_1>$ (so in our prior formulation and here, M is equivalent to Brenner et al's $<N>$). $<z_1>$ is the conventional microdosimetry specific energy deposition per charged particle traversal through a cell (ICRU 1983) and defined in Section 2.3.b of Chapter 2 - Part I. For microdosimetric hits then P(M, j) is the hit probability at a value of M in the differential range dM that the required j hits have occurred. Thus, the first term in Adaptive Response Equation (1) is the initial zero dose natural spontaneous damage with Adaptive Response reduction and the second term is the direct radiation damage [the conventional linear-quadratic behavior - ($\alpha D + \beta D^2$)] with also a possible threshold and Adaptive Response radioprotective reduction as was found to be the case in prior work. We see at zero dose, D = 0, then M = 0, PAF_S (M,N) = PAF_R (M,Q) = PAF_D (M,U) = 0 and DR = P_{spon} .

As is frequently the case for risks reported by the Radiation Effects Research Foundation for the Japanese A-bomb survivor data, we wished to express the relative risk, RR, (normalized with respect to zero radiation dose natural spontaneous risk - P_{spon}) we obtained

$$RR = DR/P_{spon} = \{ \ [\ 1 - P_{prot-s\infty} \ PAF_S \ (M,N) \ ]$$
$$+ [\ 1 - P_{prot-r\infty} \ PAF_R \ (M,Q) \ ] \ f(M) \ PAF_D \ (M,U) \ (\ \alpha D + \beta D^2 \ ) \ / \ P_{spon} \ \} \qquad (3)$$

This corresponds to the prior work Equation (16) of Leonard (2007a) and Equation (19) of Leonard (2008c). We see that for absorbed dose = D = 0, then M = 0 and RR = 1.0. BEIR VI (1999) makes use of Relative Risk in evaluating lung cancer risks as seen in Figure 1C. These Adaptive Response Microdose Model parameters are also explicitly defined in Appendix B.

2.1.b The Combined Adaptive Response and Bystander Model

We review the formulation of the composite BE and AR Microdose Model (Leonard 2008a, 2008c). The radiation dose response is expressed in terms of charged particle traversals through the exposed medium using Specific Energy Hits as the independent variable. The experimental radio-biologists conduct their experimental exposures in terms of tissue absorbed dose. However, in planning and analyzing results, the independent variable Specific Energy Hits per Nucleus is important, given by tissue absorbed dose $D / <z_1>$. We here have therefore provided, as was done in prior work, the BaD Model and our composite AR and BE Microdose Model in terms of both of these independent variables – and also, as will be seen, provide the abscissa of our graphs with both. For the composite model and the BaD Model, we have assumed that there are no intracellular interactions between the separate processes creating the potentially deleterious (or protective) Bystander and the potentially protective Adaptive Response mechanisms. The composite model encompassing both processes can be given by

Dose Response = Initial Spontaneous Damage (with AR protection) + Bystander Effect Damage (with AR protection) + Direct Deleterious Damage (with AR protection)

As defined above, the zero dose natural spontaneous damage is given by P_{spon}, as in Equation (1). Thus, from Equation (3), we have for the normalized relative risk as a function of tissue absorbed dose, RR = Dose Response / P_{spon} and

$$RR(D, N, Q, U) = [1 - P_{prot\text{-}s\infty} PAF_S (M,N)] + \sigma [1 - Exp (- \underline{k} D)] Exp (- \xi \underline{q} D) / P_{spon}$$
$$+ [1 - P_{prot\text{-}r\infty} PAF_R (M,Q)] f(M) PAF_D (M,U) (\alpha D + \beta D^2) / P_{spon} \qquad (4)$$

where $M = D / <z_1>$. Again for absorbed dose = D = 0, M = 0 and RR = 1.0. From Equation (2) of Leonard (2008a) and Equation (34) of Leonard (2008c), the BaD Model in terms of tissue absorbed dose is given by

$$TF = \gamma \underline{q} D + \sigma [1 - Exp (-\underline{k} D)] Exp (- \underline{q} D) \qquad (5)$$

In both Equations (4) and (5), the BaD Model parameters q and k are converted to dose units by $\underline{q} = q / <z_1>$ and $\underline{k} = k / <z_1>$. Note that we do not have the BaD model Direct Damage term, $\gamma \underline{q} D$, in Equation (4) since we have the linear-quadratic Direct Damage dose response term, $(\alpha D + \beta D^2)$, already in the AR portion of the composite model. Further, $<N>$ and M are equivalent such that $(D /< z_1 >) = < N >$ and M in units of charged particle tracks (hits), So the first term, $[1 - P_{prot\text{-}s\infty} PAF_S (M,N)]$, is the normalized natural spontaneous damage including reduction by Adaptive Response radioprotection; the second term, $\sigma [1 - Exp (- \underline{k} D)] Exp (- \xi \underline{q} D) / P_{spon}$, is the normalized Bystander Damage part from the BaD model and the third term, $[1 - P_{prot\text{-}r\infty}$ $PAF_R (M,Q)] PAF_D (M,U) (\alpha D + \beta D^2) / P_{spon}$, is the normalized (to the initial spontaneous level, P_{spon}) direct linear-quadratic response (deleterious Direct Damage) including Adaptive Response radioprotection of this damage (by the Poisson PAF_R function) and a possible Poisson accumulated threshold for the initiation of this direct damage (PAF_D). The N, Q and U are the specific energy thresholds for the Poisson distributed activations.

The Relative Risk, for the composite model in terms of Specific Energy Hits per Nucleus as the independent variable, is given by

$$RR(M, N, Q, U) = [1 - P_{prot-s\infty} PAF_S (M,N)] + \sigma [1 - Exp (- k M)] Exp (- \xi q M) /$$
$$P_{spon} + [1 - P_{prot-r\infty} PAF_R (M,Q)] f(M) PAF_D (M,U) [(\alpha M <z_1>) + (\beta M^2 <z_1^2>)] /$$
$$P_{spon} \tag{6}$$

Here if M = 0, then absorbed dose = D = 0 and RR = 1.0.

2.2 Properties of Adaptive Response and Bystander Effect Relative to Combined High and Low LET Exposures

In the following sections, the experimentally observed properties of Adaptive Response and data relative to combined low LET and alpha particle dose response, based on prior observations, will be summarized . From the extensive BE data available, the basic properties of BE are examined in Chapter 2 - Part I. The basic behavior of AR with respect to lung exposure from natural background and man-made low LET radiations is examined here in Appendix A.

2.2.a Examples of Adaptive Response Protection for Challenge Dose and Spontaneous Cellular Damage with low LET Priming Doses

In our microdosimetry work (Leonard 2005, 2007a, 2007b, 2008a, 2008b, 2008c), we have shown, in the Adaptive Response data of others (Azzam et al 1996, Elmore et al 2006, 2006, Ko et al 2004, 2006, Redpath et al 1987, 2001, 2003a, 2003b, Redpath and Antoniono 1998, Shadley and Wiencke 1989, Shadley and Wolff 1987, Shadley et al 1987, Wiencke et al 1986, Wolff et al 1989) for a number of cell species, that single (i.e. just one) charged particle traversals through the cell nucleus can activate AR protection. The early work of Drs. Shadley, Wiencke and Wolff and their associates studied the effects of prior priming doses on subsequent exposures to larger challenge doses for human lymphocyte cells (Wiencke et al 1986, Shadley and Wolff 1987, Shadley et al 1987, Shadley and Wiencke 1989, Wolff et al 1989).

Figure 17, Examples of Adaptive Response radio-protection from low LET priming doses for "challenge" and spontaneous cellular damage as analyzed with the AR Microdose Model

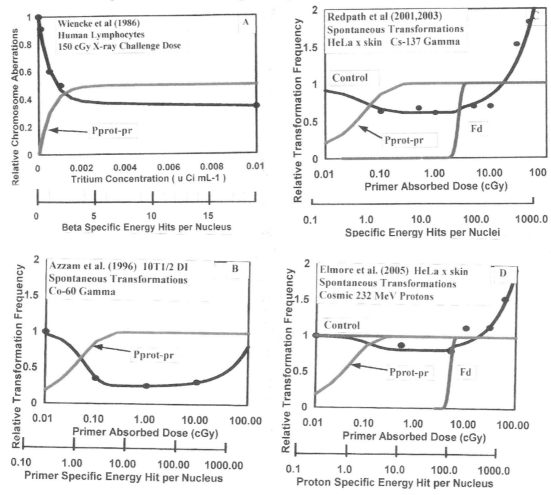

Figure 17 - Examples of Adaptive Response radio-protection from low LET priming doses for "challenge" and spontaneous cellular damage as analyzed with the AR Microdose Model (Leonard 2005, 2007a, 2007b, 2008c). Provided as red solid curves are the Poisson accumulations of single charged particle traversals (Pprot-pr) are shown to induce the protection. Specific energy hits per nucleus abscissa scales are given. Panel A – Wiencke et al (1986) data for relative chromosome aberrations in vitro versus tritiated thymidine concentrations as the primer source. Data is for a "challenge" dose of 1.5 Gy of 250 kVp X-rays. Panel B – Azzam et al (1996) Adaptive Response data for 10T1/2 cells exposed to priming doses of 60Co gamma rays producing a reduction in spontaneous neoplastic transformations. Panel C – Redpath et al (2001, 2003) Adaptive Response reduction of spontaneous transformations from exposure of HeLa x skin cells to primer doses of 137Cs gamma rays. Panel D – Elmore et al (2005) Adaptive Response reduction of spontaneous transformations from exposure of HeLa x skin cells to primer doses of 232 MeV protons.

Figure 17A provides the AR data of Wiencke et al (1996) where the human lymphocyte cells were treated with endogenic tridiated thymidine and then exposed to the exogenic 250 kVp X-rays. Shown is the fit of the AR Microdose Model showing, with the Beta Ray Specific Energy Hits per Nucleus scale, that the emission of a single low energy tritium beta ray activates the suppressive radio-protection and reduction of the cellular damage from the challenge X-rays. Relative to spontaneous AR protection, we show as Figure 17B the Adaptive Response data of Azzam et al (1996) for exposure of 10T1/2 cells to low priming doses of ^{60}Co gamma rays and subsequent reduction in the spontaneous transformation frequency. As Figure 17C, we show the AR data of Redpath and Antoniono (1998) and Redpath et al (2001) for exposure of HeLa x skin cells to low priming doses of ^{137}Cs gamma rays and, in this case, subsequent reduction in the spontaneous transformation frequency levels. The Microdose Models analysis, in these figures, shows that single radiation induced charged particle traversals through the cell nucleus initiates a Poisson accumulated AR radio-protection shown in red in the figures. This can be seen by referring to the Specific Energy Hit per Nucleus abscissa scales. As Figure 17D, we show the HeLa x skin dose response to cosmic high energy (232 MeV) protons (Elmore et al 2005). In Figure 2, it is shown, as was extensively analyzed in Leonard (2008b), that the mammogram and diagnostic X-rays extend their protection into the Bystander Damage Region (below one specific energy hit) forming a double "U" shaped dose response. The mammogram results is significant for the millions of women undergoing mammogram screening each year (Redpath 2007, Redpath and Elmore 2007, Redpath and Mitchel 2006). Altogether, the Dr. Redpath research group has shown that the Adaptive Response protection is independent of the type of low LET radiation, encompassing ^{137}Cs gamma rays, mammogram 30 kVp X-rays, diagnostic 60 kVp X-rays, ^{125}I brachytherapy photons and 232 MeV protons as well as 250 kVp X-rays (Shadley et al 1987), ^{60}Co gamma rays (Azzam et al 1996) and tritium beta rays (Wiencke et al 1986), all requiring only one charged particle traversal through the cell nucleus [see Table I, Leonard (2008b)].

2.2.b Combined Bystander Effect and Adaptive Response Effects for Low LET Radiation

As shown in Figure 18, there are now two spontaneous data sets that show that low LET radiation can active a protective Bystander behavior i.e. a reduction at very low doses where the dose is too low for even single charged particle traversals to have occurred.

Figure 18, Examples of both protective bystander and Adaptive Response radio-protection reduction in spontaneous neoplastic transformations

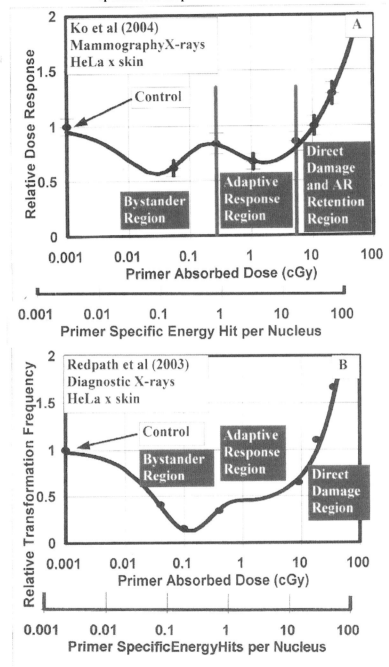

Figure 18 - Examples of both protective bystander and Adaptive Response radio-protection reduction in spontaneous neoplastic transformations. Panel A – Exposure of HeLa x skin cells to 28 kVp mammogram X-rays. Panel B – Exposure of HeLa x skin cells to 60 kVp diagnostic X-rays.

This is for both the mammogram (Ko et al 2004) mentioned above and also diagnostic (Redpath et al 2003) X-rays for HeLa x skin cells as analyzed with the Microdose Model (Leonard 2008b). It may be that the other radiations AR data for HeLa x skin would have shown protective Bystander Effect but the exposure levels of the dose sets were not low enough to encompass the Bystander Damage Region (see again Table 1, Leonard 2008b). Figure 18A and 18B provides these mammogram and diagnostic X-ray data showing the reduction in dose response at specific energy hit levels below one traversal (hit) per cell nucleus (thus protective Bystander behavior).

2.2.c Low LET Adaptive Response Radio-protection for High LET Alpha Induced Bystander Damage

The alpha particle microbeam research, primarily at the Columbia University Microbeam Facility (Randers-Pehrson et al 2001), has shown that alpha particles can induce damage to neighbor Bystander cells. The analysis presented here in Chapter 2 - Part I conclusively bears this evidence. Recent measurements have shown the range of the Bystander signal from alpha particles in three dimensional tissue is on the order of 200 μm, which would extend over many lung bronchial and bronchiolar neighbor cell diameters (Belyakov et al 2005, Leonard 2009). Of fundamental interest is whether the Bystander damage, thus known to occur in the lung, can be modulated by Adaptive Response induction with accompanying low LET radiation. Zhou et al (2003, 2004) performed micro-beam alpha particle exposures where 10% of the A_L cells were irradiated with one alpha particle. A significant Bystander damage was observed. As a second experiment, 4 hours prior to alpha irradiation, the cells were subjected to broad-beam exposures of low priming doses of 250 kVp X-rays.

Figure 19, Examples of Adaptive Response reduction of alpha particle cellular damage from priming doses of low dose radiations

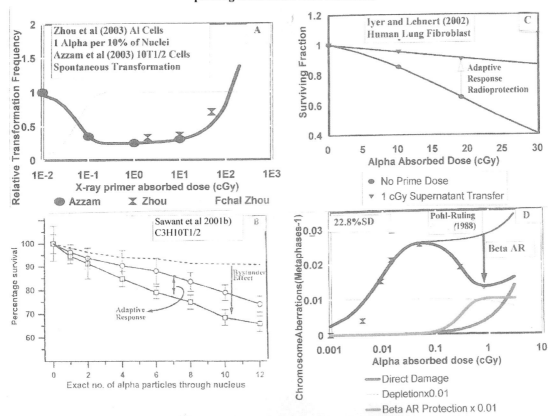

Figure 19 - Examples of Adaptive Response reduction of alpha particle cellular damage from priming doses of low dose radiations. Panel A – Shown are the data of Zhou et al (2003) from their study of Adaptive Response effects on the microbeam induced bystander damage to 10% of 10T1/2 cells. The bystander damage was normalized to damage without priming dose X-rays. We show the reduction of the bystander damage from priming doses of X-rays. Shown also as a comparison is the data of Azzam et al (1996) presented in Figure 4B. Panel B – The surviving fraction data of Sawant et al (2001) for injection of specific numbers of alpha particles, showing a reduction in cell killing for C3H 10T1/2 cells when pre-exposed to X-rays. Panel C – The results of Iyer and Lehnert (2002) alpha particle exposures where prior exposure of super-nutrients to X-rays produces reduction in alpha particle human lung fibroblast cell killing. Panel D – The Pohl-Ruling (1983, 1988) non-monotonic dose response of chromosome aberrations in human lymphocytes from radon alpha particles, caused by Adaptive Response radio-protection from radon progeny beta rays. Reproduced from Leonard (2008a) with permission.

Figure 19A shows the relative response and approximately a 75% reduction in the Bystander damage from the alpha irradiations induced by the low LET X-rays. We also show in Figure 19A the Azzam et al (1996) AR data for ^{60}Co priming dose exposures, as a comparison, showing nearly the same large magnitude of AR protection. Again with the micro-beam facility, Sawant et al (2001a) injected exact numbers of alpha particles through the nuclei of 10% of the C3H 10T1/2 cell population and measured the clonal survival. As a second experiment, they exposed all the cells to a broad-beam exposure of

2 cGy of 250 kVp X-rays prior to the microbeam alpha exposures. Figure 19B provides the percent survival data showing about a 50% Adaptive Response reduction in cell killing from the priming dose AR protection.

In the medium transfer experiment of Iyer and Lehnert (2002) the surviving fraction was measured for the exposure of human lung fibroblast to radon alpha particles. As the second experiment, they exposed supernatant medium to 1 cGy of X-rays and then transferred to the *in vitro* culture before alpha irradiation. As seen in Figure 3C, what was observed was a very large reduction in cell killing even greater than that observed by Sawant et al (2001b).

A study was conducted by Wolff et al (1991) to examine the effectiveness of 250 kVp X-rays in inducing Adaptive Response radio-protection for challenge doses of radon alpha particles in human lymphocyte cells. Cells were exposed to a dose of 16.4 cGy of radon alphas alone. In a second experiment, the cells were first exposed to 2 cGy of X-rays and then 15.3 cGy of radon alphas. A 51% decrease in the yield of chromosome aberrations was observed.

We had mentioned in our earlier work, the possibility that the human lymphocyte exposures of Pohl-Ruling (1988) to radon alpha particles may have exhibited a combination Bystander Effect and an Adaptive Response modulation in the plateau region of her observed dose response curve (see Figure 4, Leonard 2007a). In our more recent work (see Figure 4, Leonard 2008a), her data was fitted to the Bystander BaD Model but the model was unable to justify the depth of the "U" shaped plateau response. This in contrast to excellent fits for the data considered in Part I (Leonard et al 2009a) and the other Bystander data examined in Leonard (2008a). A detailed analysis of the Pohl-Ruling data and progeny beta activation of Adaptive Response is given in Leonard (2008a). In considering the 8 different energy beta rays emitted in the ^{222}Rn decay chain, it was found that enough beta radiation was present for at least one beta traversal per human lymphocyte cell nucleus in the higher radon plateau region. Figure 3D shows the magnitude of the Adaptive Response reduction to produce the non-monotonic behavior "U" shaped dose response. For the Pohl-Ruling data, the radon alpha damage may thus be considered a "challenge" dose behavior and the accompanying radon progeny betas considered a primer to induce AR protection but with the beta "priming" dose increasing along with the radon progeny "challenge" alpha dose until just enough beta ray traversals occur to induce adaptive response. This implies that human lung tissue may be subjected

66

to Adaptive Response reduction in lung cancer risk from the radon progeny own beta radiation that may dominate over the Bystander chromosome damage. We will consider these radon progeny betas as one low LET radiation source of adaptive protection against lung cancer in later Section 3.1.e.

2.2.d *The Time Dependent Behavior of Adaptive Response Radio-protection – Fading and Dose Rate Effects*

Shadley and Wiencke (1989) studied the sensitivity of Adaptive Response protection with respect to the dose rate of the priming dose for challenge dose experiments with human lymphocytes using 250 kVp X-rays. In evaluating their data, it was found that there is a dose rate threshold as well as a single traversal dose threshold (Leonard 2005, 2007b). Elmore et al (2006) measured the dose rate behavior of Adaptive Response for spontaneous damage in HeLa x skin cells, which we examined with the Microdose Model in Section 3.1 of Leonard (2008c) with again a dose rate threshold being required to model the data. Shadley et al (1987) varied the time between the administration of the priming dose and the later challenge dose. It had been known from others that the endogenic cellular activation of the AR radio-protection required 4 to 6 hours.

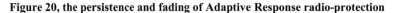

Figure 20, the persistence and fading of Adaptive Response radio-protection

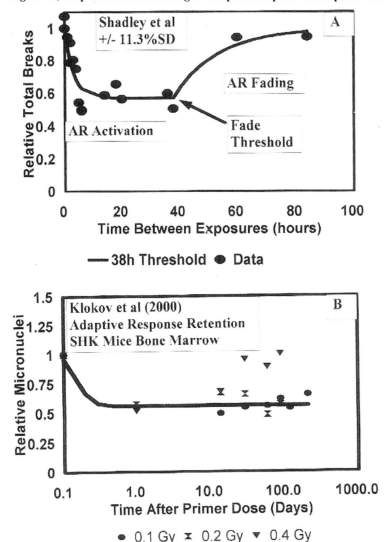

Figure 20 - The persistence and fading of Adaptive Response radio-protection. Panel A – From Shadley et al (1987). The normalized reduction in relative chromosome breaks as a function of delay time between administering of the 1.5 Gy X-ray "challenge" dose after the 1.0 cGy primer dose. The AR protection is shown to materialize in about 4-6 hours and is sustained for about 38 hours before fading and completely dissipating. Panel B – The data of Klokov et al (2000) showing reduction of mice bone marrow micronuclei after exposure in vivo to X-rays as a function of time after exposure. Both reproduced from Leonard (2007b) with permission.

From Leonard (2007b), we reproduce the Figure 1C graph as Figure 20A here of the Adaptive Response protection afforded the challenge dose as a function of time between the priming dose and the challenge dose. It is shown that the protection is maintained at a constant level up to 38 hours but then begins to fade and the protection is dissipated. The cell cycle time for human lymphocytes is approximately 38 hours. Considering the dose rate threshold also being compatible with the cell cycle time, the data suggests that the protection may be lost at mitosis although this has not been conclusively confirmed in the laboratory. The fact that after the AR activation threshold and Poisson transition of the AR protection, the protection remains constant as primer dose is increased (as seen in Figure 20A) suggests that early stages of the cell cycle may be insensitive to AR activation and the magnitude of the protection, when it becomes fully effective, is related to the fraction of time in the entire cell cycle that the cell is sensitive to the single charged particle traversal that produces the activation. Other data however contradict the mitosis AR dissipation hypothesis. Klokov et al (2000) found that exposure of the SHK mice *in vivo* to low doses between 0.1 and 0.4 Gy produced a reduction in bone marrow micronuclei that was sustained for up to 100 days. We show their data as Figure 20B. We will discuss other very recent data, primarily from Dr. Ron Mitchels research group (Mitchel et al 1999, 2002, 2003, 2004, Mitchel 2006, 2007a, 2007b, 2008), showing the persistence of AR effects *in vivo* for much longer times in the later Discussion sections of Part III (Leonard et al 2009b). It may be that AR is sustained longer *in vivo* than in tissue cultures where immortalized cells are used.

2.2.e The Dose Region of the Dose Response Curve for the Adaptive Response Radio-protection to be Effective

We have divided the basic dose response curve into three regions i.e. the Bystander Damage Region, the Adaptive Response Region and the Direct Damage Region as shown in Figure 18. Of significant interest is the questions of "at what dose level does the AR protection begin and at what dose level does the deleterious Direct Damage begin to dominate over the protection and also what role does the quality of the radiation plays?". The dose region of low LET radiation exposures, where humans may expect Adaptive Response radio-protection, depends on the size of the energy deposition for the single specific energy hits that are found to first begin to activate AR.

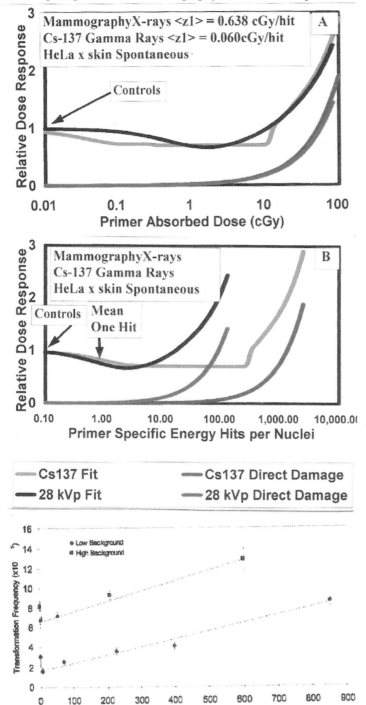

Figure 21 - Comparing the Ko et al mammography data and the Redpath et al 137Cs data. Panel A – the simultaneous plot of the two data sets and Microdose Model fits as a function of Primer Absorbed Dose. We see that the two high dose Direct Damage curves very nearly coincide even though the LET's and <z1> values are very different, indicating the total energy deposited to the cells dictates the priming dose induced high dose Direct Damage response, not the Specific Energy for each hit. Panel B – Plot of the data and fits as a function of accumulated Primer Specific Energy Hits per Nuclei. We see that, as

determined from our Microdose Model analysis, that a Poisson distributed mean of one single Specific Energy Hit activates the Adaptive Response protection. This means that Adaptive Response activation is solely dependent on a single Specific Energy Hit regardless of the size of the energy in the deposition and independent of the Primer Absorbed Dose. Panels A and B reproduced from Leonard (2008b) with permission. Panel C – Reproduction of Redpath and Elmore (2007) Figure 1 with permission. Analysis of their combined data for 137Cs gamma rays, 28 kVp X-rays, 60 kVp X-rays, 232 MeV protons (Redpath et al 2001, Redpath et al 2003, Ko et al 2004, Elmore et al 2005) showing a threshold and linearity of the Direct Damage dose response. Shown also is an apparent retention of the AR protection in the Direct Damage Region.

Mitchel (2010) has examined the range of dose where AR is effective. He notes that there is an upper detrimental threshold and a lower threshold below which AR protection is absent. His typical range is estimated to be between 1 and 100 mGy. To examine here what factors influence the AR range and what determines the thresholds, we have compared (see Figure 4, Leonard 2008b) the AR behavior of HeLa x skin cells for ^{137}Cs 0.66 MeV gamma rays and the much lower energy 28 kVp mammogram X-rays in Figure 21. In this earlier work, we examined the differences in the initiations of the Adaptive Response radio-protections and the beginning of the Direct Damage domination at higher doses. One question was "At what dose or charged particle traversals does the Direct Damage begin to dominate over the AR protection?" In Figure 21A, the abscissa scale is in units of Primer Absorbed Dose where we show for both radiations that the Direct Damage component begins to dominate at a threshold of about 10 cGy but the lower dose thresholds for AR activation is quite different for the two radiations, in terms of dose. In Figure 21B, we use Primer Specific Energy Hits per Nucleus as the abscissa scale and we see that the lower dose AR thresholds coincide at a mean of one specific energy hit per nucleus, as first stated in Leonard (2005), but the beginning of the Direct Damage component is over a factor of 10 different in terms of hits. This is because the respective values of $<z_1>$ (which determines the AR single hit threshold) are quite different i.e. 0.638 cGy/hit and 0.050 cGy/hit for the mammogram X-rays and the ^{137}Cs gamma rays respectively. We have found that the constancy of the Direct Damage threshold persists, in terms of dose, for the other radiations used by Dr. Redpaths group. In fact, Redpath et al (2007) showed this to be true in analyzing the dose response slopes of their different results for high and low spontaneous level AR experiments. We reproduce their Figure 1 as Panel C of Figure 21. This means that the dose range for the AR protection is shorter for radiations with higher $<z_1>$ value i.e. lower energy radiations, with correspondingly higher LETs. No data has shown Adaptive Response radio-protection being induced by naturally occurring alpha particle radiations, the lack

71

of this then as evidenced from our Part I analysis. This may be because the $<z_1>$ values for alpha particles range from about 200 to 400 mGy/hit – in the region for the Direct Damage threshold, negating any observable evidence of AR by domination of the Direct Damage which is found to begin between 10 and 100 mGy deposition to the cell as shown in Figure 21. Thus we would not expect any Adaptive Response dose response protection since the alpha damage is so severe. Feinendegen et al (2010) discuss this and provides $<z_1>$ values in their Table 1 for common radiations and showing a $<z_1>$ for 4 MeV alpha particles of 350 mGy per hit. As we have shown in Chapter 2, Section 2.3.b, $<z_1>$ depends on the size of the "target" cell as well as the LET of the radiation. Table I of Leonard (2007a) provides some values of $<z_1>$ for the low LET radiations for the cell species analyzed there. The exposures in Figure 2 are for relatively high dose rates and would not reveal any dose rate effects eluded to by Dr. Mitchel.

2.2.f The Potential Retention of the Adaptive Response Radio-protection at High Dose Levels in the Direct Damage Region.

Microdose Model analysis of dose response data have shown that a threshold seems to exist for the induction of the Direct Damage as dose increases when AR protection is present. Some data also show that the Adaptive Response protection is retained at the higher doses above the Direct Damage threshold. This has been examined in Figure 1D, 2 and 3C of Leonard (2008b). AR retention is seen to occur if, by extrapolation of the Direct Damage, linear- quadratic, region back to the origin of the dose response curve, the extrapolation intersects below the zero dose spontaneous level. The Figure 21C here of Redpath et al shows an extrapolation well below the spontaneous level for all their AR data, thus showing AR retention even at doses where the Direct Damage dominates.

2.3 The Human Lung Cells as "Targets" for Low LET Traversals and Subsequent Energy Depositions per Traversal

2.3.a The Size of the Human Lung Target Cells Susceptible to Carcinogenesis

Section 2.3.a of Part I discusses the estimated size of the three lung "target" cell species susceptible to carcinogenesis. They are the bronchial basal, bronchial secretory and bronchiolar secretory lung cells and each vary in size and hence present different target sizes for radiation "Hits" for the radon progeny alpha particles and the low LET

AR inducing radiations. This thus affects the value of $<z_1>$ and cell hit rates relative the exposure doses. For our analysis. we estimate the three cell diameters to be 9.0, 17.7 and 10.7 μm for the bronchial basal, bronchial secretory and the bronchiolar secretory cells, respectively. These are in agreement with the BEIR VI Table 2-1 data and the same data used by Little and Wakeford (2001). We use these diameters in Tables A1, A2 and A3 of Appendix A to estimate the Specific Energy Deposition per Nucleus Traversals for the low LET radiations received by the lung from human exposures at the UNSCEAR world average low LET human exposure levels (Table 1 herein).

2.3.b Method for Determination of the Mean Specific Energy per Sensitive Volume Hit - $<z_1>$

Section 2.3.b of Chapter 2 - Part I provides the means to determine the microdose parameter Specific Energy Deposition per Charged Particle Traversal, $<z_1>$. It is dependent on the linear energy transfer, Le (in units of keV / μm) and the mean chord length, ∫ (in units of μm), traversed through the sensitive volume. As was the case in the earlier works (Leonard 2005, 2007a, 2007b, 2008a, 2008b, 2008c) the sensitive volume here is chosen to be the nucleus for the three human lung cell species. BEIR VI (1999) and James et al (2004) in their analysis with respect to alpha particle traversals consider the nucleus as the sensitive region for lung cancer induction. We noted in Section 2.3.a of Part I, by considering the mean chord length per cell cross-section area, an analytical approximation for $<z_1>$ was offered by Kellerer and Rossi (1972) as a function of spherical critical volume diameter, d, and the linear energy transfer, Le, of the radiation, i.e.

$$<z_1> = 22.95(\text{cGy g keV}^{-1} / \text{chord length-μm})\text{Le} / \rho \, d^2 \text{ cGy / Hit (nucleus traversal)} \quad (7)$$

where ρ = density of cell tissue.

As we have stated. we estimate the accuracy in determining the cell nucleus diameters to be about ± 20 %SD and the overall accuracy of $<z_1>$ to be ± 30 %SD due to uncertainties in Le also. The impact of this on the use of the model is addressed in Leonard (2008c).

2.4 The Methods for Assessing the Combined Influence of the Bystander Effect and Adaptive Response on Human Lung Cancer Risks

1. We have shown in Section 2.2.a above that all types of low LET ionizing radiations will activate the Adaptive Response radio-protection within cells, from single charged particle traversals through the nucleus. To evaluate the effect of natural background and man-made radiations on Adaptive Response radio-protection of humans, it is necessary to identify all the low LET whole body radiations and amount of dose from each to lung tissue.

2. To determine the charged particle track accumulation in the lung tissue, we will evaluate the new knowledge that has been gained about both a.) the Bystander Effect and general cellular response to alpha particle radiation in Chapter 2 - Part I and b.) the protective behavior of Adaptive Response as reviewed here in the above Section 2.2. As was done in the recent prior works (Leonard 2008a, 2008b, 2008c), we will use the composite Adaptive Response and Bystander Effect Microdose Model, presented in detail in Leonard (2008c) and reviewed above, to examine and evaluate the expected behavior in the human lung.

With the Microdose Model, we have found that Adaptive Response has the very specific behavior, in particular, that single cell low LET charged particle traversals activates the protection and the protection results in between 50 and 80% reduction in potentially carcinogenic radiation induced exogenic cellular damage and endogenic spontaneous cellular damage. The protection is afforded for alpha particle cell damage as well as low LET radiation cell damage as shown in Section 2.2.c. The protection is relatively independent of the type of priming dose radiation quality, encompassing low and high energy X-rays, beta rays, gamma rays and even high energy cosmic protons. We have seen in Section 2.2.e that, at higher doses, the protection may be retained but at about 10 cGy of exposure the excessive damage from the priming dose begins to dominate. In Section 2.2.d that the duration of the protection, from dose rate and fading studies, is at least through one cell mitotic cycle and thus we will evaluate the charged particle traversals to the lung cells for the 30 day mitotic cycle (James et al 2004).

3. RESULTS

3.1 General Approach to Assessment

A fundamental unknown, at the time the BEIR VI (1999) report was drafted was the amount of influence Adaptive Response has on radon progeny alpha particle initiation of human lung cancer. We here endeavor to assess the magnitude of Adaptive Response radio-protection that humans receive from the various low LET radiations received by humans on a routine, day-to-day basis. Based on the extensive supportive data, some of which is presented in the prior sections, we assume that single radiation induced charged particle traversals activates the Poisson transition of each traversed cell to the Adaptive Response radio-protective state. In Appendix A, we first tabulated the low LET radiations that an average person would receive using the United Nations worldwide average values for each of the radiation components. The UNSCEAR (2000) worldwide human exposures are provided in Table 1.

Table 2, UNSCEAR (2000) Estimated Worldwide Annual Human Radiation Exposure

Table 2 - UNSCEAR (2000) ESTIMATED WORLDWIDE ANNUAL HUMAN RADIATION EXPOSURE

Average radiation dose from natural sources

Source	Worldwide average annual effective dose (mSv)	Typical range (mSv)
External exposure		
Cosmic rays	0.4	0.3-1.0 [a]
Terrestrial gamma rays	0.5	0.3-0.6 [b]
Internal exposure		
Inhalation (mainly radon)	1.2	0.2-10 [c]
Ingestion	0.3	0.2-0.8 [d]
Total	2.4	1-10

a Range from sea level to high ground elevation.
b Depending on radionuclide composition of soil and building materials.
c Depending on indoor accumulation of radon gas.
d Depending on radionuclide composition of foods and drinking water.

Radiation exposures from diagnostic medical x-ray examinations

Health care level	Population per physician	Annual number of examinations per 1,000 population	Average annual effective dose to population (mSv)
I	<1 000	920	1.2
II	1 000-3 000	150	0.14
III	3 000-10 000	20	0.02
IV	>10 000	<20	<0.02
Worldwide average		330	0.4

Average external radiation doses from terrestrial radiation components - UNSCEAR (2000)

Source	Worldwide average annual effective tissue absorbed dose (mGy)	Typical range (mGy)
Uranium series isotopes gamma rays	0.122	0.073 - 0.146
Thorium series isotopes gamma rays	0.195	0.117 - 0.234
Potassium-40 gamma rays	0.183	0.110 - 0.220
Total	0.500	0.300 - 0.600

In Table A1 of Part II - Appendix A, the radiations are listed with the energies, fraction of decays and the LETs for each radiation component (Attix 1986). As was explained above, to obtain the number of charged particle traversals, the Specific Energy Deposition per Traversal, $<z_1>$, is required. In Section 2.3.b, using Equation (7), it is shown that the diameter of the "target" cell as well as the LET of the radiation is needed. In Table A2, the LETs and the cell diameters of the three sensitive lung cells, bronchial basal, bronchial secretory and bronchiolar secretory, are given. In Table A2, using the UNSCEAR human exposure levels and the calculated $<z_1>$ values for each natural background and man-made radiation component is tabulated. The number of cell traversals (hits) occurring in one cell cycle (30 days) is then tabulated as a final result. These are for the worldwide annual average low LET radiations, giving traversals per 30 day cell cycles, and at the median radon concentration of 24.3 Bq m^{-3}. In Table A2, we find that a significant fraction of the lung cells are traversed by single low LET charged particles and a sizable Adaptive Response radio-protection must be present i.e. 28.6%, 72.9% and 37.9% in the three respective cells.

We are interested in evaluating the magnitude of the AR protection as a function of varying human radon exposure and varying low LET human exposures. As noted, there are two lung dose components that vary with radon concentration. They are 1.) the radon progeny beta ray dose to the lung, that varies linearly with radon concentration and 2.) the terrestrial Uranium gamma ray dose which we have evaluated from USGS data and some indoor gamma ray measurements and presented in the following sections. By conservatively assuming the other human exposure components remain at the worldwide averages, we have estimated the variation in lung cell traversals with increasing radon concentration. As Table A3, we show a section (for Basal lung cells) of the spread sheet used to tabulate the Specific Energy Hits to the lung cells as a function of increasing radon concentration.

3.2 Effectiveness of Low LET Radiations in Providing Single Charged Particle Traversals to Lung Tissue

Humans receive a substantial amount of low LET ionizing radiations from natural background and man-made radiation sources. In Section 2.2, we have cited numerous radio-biology data showing that cells undergo a hormesis type Adaptive Response protective behavior from very low doses of low LET radiation. It has been shown that single, radiation induced, charged particle traversals through the cell nucleus activates this AR protection. It has also been shown that beta rays, X-rays and gamma rays seem to be equally effective in inducing this AR protection. This is substantiated by the low energy, 0.0186 MeV tritium beta AR data of Wiencke et al (1986), the 28 kVp X-ray AR data of Ko et al (2004), the 60 kVp diagnostic X-ray AR data of Redpath et al (2003), the 250 kVp X-rays AR data of Shadley et al (1987), the 31-35 keV photons ^{125}I brachytherapy AR data of Elmore et al (2006), the 0.66 MeV ^{137}Cs gamma ray AR data of Redpath et al (2001), the 1.17-1.33 MeV ^{60}Co gamma ray AR data of Azzam et al (1996) and the cosmic ray level 232 MeV proton AR data of Elmore et al (2005). The range of low LET values that span these radiation sources is from about 0.1 to 2.0

keV/μm and the range of Specific Energy Depositions per Cell Nucleus Traversal, $<z_1>$, is from about 0.02 to about 1.0 cGy/hit. The transmission range in tissue is from about 0.01 to 1.0 cm and therefore a 1 MeV photon produced electron or a beta ray will traverse many cell diameters compared to the μm range alpha particles in tissue. Figure 2-1 of BEIR VI illustrates the large difference in tracks for 1 Gy of low LET tracks (1000 tracks) to high LET alpha particles (4 tracks).

Figure 22, Radiation Penetrations and Transmissions Through Tissues

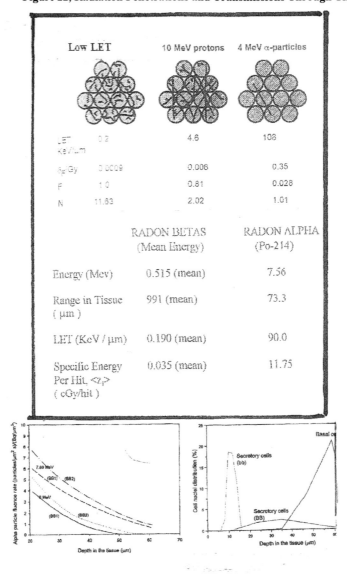

Figure 22 - Top Panel - Graphics showing the difference in tissue interactions of low LET radiation induced charged particles and high LET alpha particles. Bottom Panels – Left, Alpha particle fluence as a function of distance through human lung tissue. Right, Location of basal and secretory cells depth in human lung tissue.

We provide as Figure 22, a chart relative to beta or photon producing electrons and alpha traversals. Shown in the upper section are the effects from low LET radiation, 10 MeV protons and 4 Mev alpha particles in terms of LET and number of cells traversed. In the lower section, specifically for radon progeny beta rays and the 7.69 MeV ^{214}Po radon progeny alphas, we give the range in tissue, the LET and $<z_1>$ showing a considerably lower dose of the radon progeny beta rays is capable of delivering the necessary single charged particle traversal to the lung cells to induce AR protection against chromosome damage inducing lung cancer. The radon progeny are deposited on the interior lung air passage surfaces, and become located primarily in the mucous gel and cilia regions [see Figures 9-2 through 9-5 of NRC (1991)]. In the lower two panels of Figure 22, we reproduce graphs of Nikezic and Yu (2001) that show the relative location of the basal and secretory cells relative to the radon progeny. The average alpha particle emitted from the progeny is attenuated by at least 50% before reaching the three cancer sensitive cells. The attenuation of the progeny beta rays is negligible. Strictly from an energy deposition basis, the total beta disintegration energy is 2.12 MeV, from Figure A2 and Table A1. The total energy of the two alpha particles is 6.00 + 7.69 = 13.69 MeV. If 50% is lost by attenuation then the deposition energy of the betas to the target cells is about 31%. Thus the progeny beta rays contribute a significant amount of low LET radiation, and potential Adaptive Response protection, to the sensitive lung tissue.

3.3 Properties, Magnitudes and Variations of Radiation Sources to Humans

3.3.a Sources of Low LET Radiations Experienced by Humans

In Table 1 and Section 3.3.a.1 below, we identify the various components to the radiations received by humans, for the purpose of assessing the AR inducing low LET radiations to the human lung that can activate Adaptive Response radio-protection to the lung cells and affect the risk probabilities of human lung cancer from radon progeny alpha particles. We then, in Appendix A, used the United Nations world-wide average exposure rates (UNSCEAR 2000) of these low LET components, given in Table 1, to estimate the low LET charged particle traversals to the three most sensitive lung cells i.e. bronchial basal, bronchial secretory and bronchiolar secretory cells, for potential AR activation. Then the special effects like the statistical distributions of these world-wide averages, from variations in geological and ecological conditions, are considered with

79

respect to a high and low range of human exposure to these AR inducing charged particle traversals. The variations of U series terrestrial dose and beta radon progeny dose with radon indoor concentration are considered.

3.3.a.1 World-wide Averages of Human Low LET Exposures

Americans receive a population averaged annual dose equivalent of about 2.4 mSv of background radiation of which 39 % is low LET, consisting primarily of about 20% terrestrial gamma rays, 12% a cosmic ray component and 7% internal (ingestion) component, and 52 % from high LET radon progeny (BEIR VII 2006). We also receive an annual average of about 0.5 mSv of man-made radiation, of which at least 98 % is low LET. Thus, the major components of our total population averaged annual dose of 2.9 mSv is about 1.44 mSv low LET and about 1.25 mSv high LET radon progeny alphas. The United Nations Scientific Committee on the Effects of Atomic Radiation (UNSCEAR 2000) provides slightly different values for world-wide averaged human exposures and provides a more detailed break-down of the various components (summarized in Table 1). They estimate the external exposure from cosmic rays to be 0.3 mSv for the directly ionizing component and 0.055 mSv for cosmic neutrons. The internal cosmogenic dose is about 0.010 mSv. From external natural radioactivity exposure, they estimate 0.15 mSv for ^{40}K, 0.100 mSv for the ^{238}U series and 0.160 mSv from the ^{232}Th series. Internal exposure from ingestion of radio-isotopes is estimated to be about 0.18 mSv from potassium-40, 0.006 from ^{87}Rb, 0.005 mSv from ^{238}U transition to ^{234}U, 0.007 mSv for ^{230}Th, 0.007 from ^{226}Ra, 0.12 mSv from ^{210}Pb transition to ^{210}Po, 0.003 from ^{232}Th, and 0.013 from ^{228}Ra to ^{224}Ra. The total annual exposure from natural sources equals about 0.765 mSv external and 0.356 mSv internal. UNSCEAR estimates that humans receive about 0.4 mSv from diagnostic medical exposures. Rounded off UNSCEAR values for the net components are in their report to the UN General assembly are external cosmic rays 0.2 mSv, external terrestrial gamma rays 0.5 mSv, medical 0.4 mSv, internal ingestion 0.3 mSv and inhalation 1.2 mSv of which 1.1 mSv is considered radon (with a US median of 24.3 Bq m^{-3} concentration). Then the non-radon human exposures, which would be about 99% low LET, is 1.7 mSv per year. There are special considerations relative to the terrestrial radiations with respect to the relative contributions of the three components, Uranium series, Thorium series and Potassium-40 and their indoor distributions. Also, it is known that there is a correlation between the indoor radon concentration and the Uranium series indoor component, which we will

80

address in the next section. Further, as we showed for the Pohl-Ruling data in Figure 2D and evaluated by Jostes et al (1991), the beta ray dose from the lung deposited radon progeny contributes a significant number of lung cell low LET charged particle traversals that increases with increase in radon concentration. So the world-wide averages for U series dose and progeny beta dose is coupled to the world-wide variation in indoor radon concentration.

3.3.b Special Consideration for Terrestrial Radiation Components and Distributions.

3.3.b.1 Local Variations - USGS and EPA Terrestrial Gamma and Radon Concentrations

We next examine the variability of the human exposures worldwide using the UNSCEAR maximum and minimum range values in Table 1. In quoting US or world-wide averages for human exposure to ionizing radiations, usually a statistical range is also given, for example by BEIR VII and UNSCEAR. More specific data are provided by the United States Geological Service (USGS) for the US lower 48 states (Duval et al 2005, Phillips et al 1993). An extensive program of mapping the terrestrial radiation components, U, Th and ^{40}K exposures at 1 meter above ground level has been completed using highly sensitive aerial radiation monitoring equipment. Details relative to the airborne gamma ray method are found in a NOAA report (NOAA 2008), a DOE report (DOE 2002) and Schwartz et al (1993).

Figure 23, Reproduction of USGS terrestrial radiation maps

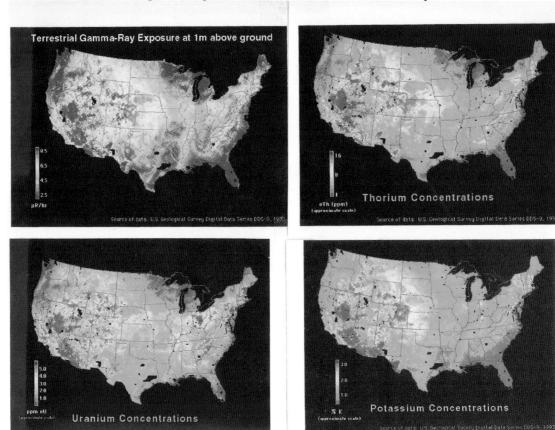

Figure 23 – Reproduction of USGS terrestrial radiation maps (Duval et al 1989) for total gamma ray exposure and separate exposures from Uranium series, Thorium series and Potassium-40.

Figure 23 provides four maps of the terrestrial Gamma-Ray Exposure at 1 meter above ground. The first panel shows the net from all three gamma ray sources in units of μR/h (1 R = 1 Roentgen = 0.86 Rad = 0.86 cGy). The other three maps show the gamma radiation levels for Uranium, Thorium and ^{40}K. The units for U and Th are parts per million (ppm) and for ^{40}K are %K. To obtain the exposure dose rates for each and total, the USGS conversion equation is

Total Exposure Rate (nGy/h) = 13.2 (nGy/h per %K) K (%K) + 5.48 (nGy/h per ppm U) U (ppm) + 2.72 (nGy/h per ppm Th) Th (ppm)   (8)

We show the gamma ray spectra for the three components as Figure A1 of Appendix A. It is seen that the South-west region of the US shows the major gamma ray exposure for all three components. The Pacific North-west and Florida are seen to be the lowest terrestrial gamma ray exposure regions. Digital reports have been issued by USGS presently for only the Uranium series gamma ray dose data (in ppm) by counties for all states.

Figure 24, Reproduction of EPA radon maps (EPA 2003)

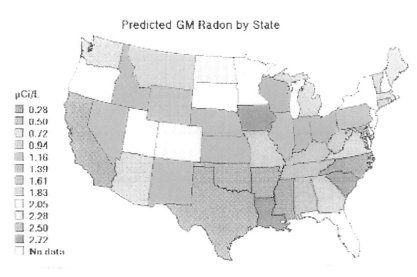

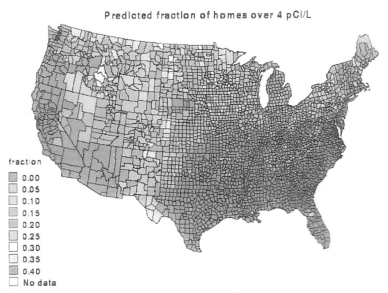

Figure 24 - Reproduction of EPA radon maps (EPA 2003) showing indoor radon levels by states and by counties.

EPA (2003) distributed maps are available for geometric mean radon levels in the US, also. We show as Figure 24A, a map of the geometric mean residential radon concentrations by states in pCi/L units. As Figure 24B, we provide a map of the US showing by county the mean residential radon levels in fractions of homes over 4 pCi/L. The EPA High-Radon Project has also provided in Excell spread sheet format itemized data on individual radon measurements organized by counties in each state.

3.3.b.2 Local Variations - Special Measurements of Radon and Gamma Ray Distributions

Relative to the distribution of the terrestrial gamma ray exposures, the state of California has been mapped and digital data provided by county has been provided (Wollenberg et al 1994).

Figure 25, Analysis of the terrestrial gamma ray data of Woolenberg et al (1995) for the state of California

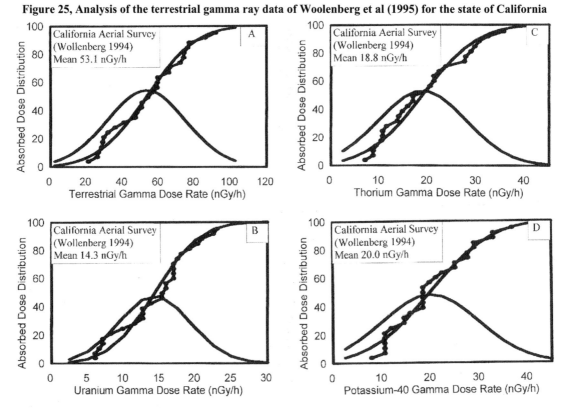

Figure 25 - Analysis of the terrestrial gamma ray data of Woolenberg et al (1995) for the state of California by counties providing Normal Distribution for each component and the geometric mean averages. Panel A – Total gamma ray. Panel B – Uranium series gamma ray. Panel C – Thorium gamma ray. Panel D – Potassium-40 gamma ray.

We have analyzed the distributions of the U, Th and ⁴⁰K county data and provide these as Figure 25. The average total terrestrial gamma ray dose rate in California is 53.1 nGy/h. The respective gamma ray dose rates for the three components, U, Th and ⁴⁰K, are 14.3, 18.8 and 20.0 nGy/h. The data has been fit to Normal Distribution functions with σ's of 5, 9, and 9.9 nGy/h and standard errors of 0.8, 0.9 and 1.0 nGy/h, respectively. From another part of the world, Clouvas et al (2001) have preformed detailed indoor radiation measurements in over 1000 Greek homes. They used a high resolution Germanium gamma ray detector system to resolve the separate gamma rays from the Uranium, Thorium and Potassium isotopes.

Figure 26, Analysis of the frequency distribution data of Chouvas et al (2001) for residual terrestrial gamma ray exposure

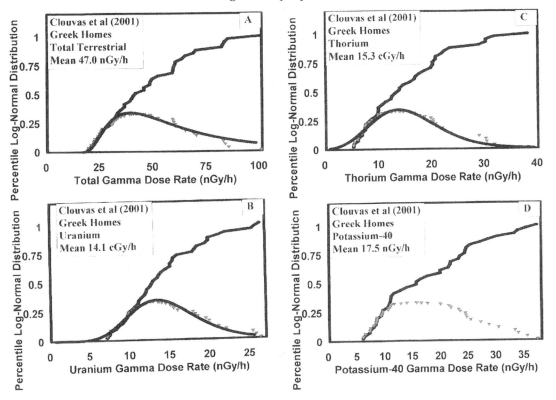

Figure 26 – Analysis of the frequency distribution data of Chouvas et al (2001) for residential terrestrial gamma ray exposure showing Log-Normal Distribution and mean values. Panel A – Total gamma ray. Panel B – Uranium series gamma ray. Panel C – Thorium gamma ray. Panel D – Potassium-40 gamma ray.

Figure 26 provides their dose rate distributions for the U, Th and K sources. We have best fitted the data more accurately to log-normal distributions than a normal distribution, however the Potassium data showed a distribution between a normal and a log-normal. The total mean gamma dose rate was 47.0 nGy/h. The three components dose rates were 14.1, 15.3 and 17.5 nGy/h for U, Th and K respectively.

Clouvas et al (2006) recently performed a new survey of Greek homes where both indoor gamma ray dose rates and radon concentrations were measured. In a total of 311 homes, the total gamma ray dose rate was 58.33 ±12.15 nGy/h and the three components were 14.61 ±3.80 (U), 20.81 ± 3.78 (Th) and 22.92 ± 4.92 (K) nGy/h. The average radon concentration was 34 Bq m^{-3}.

Figure 27, Analysis of separate data by Clouvas et al (2001) showing indoor gamma ray does rates and indoor radon concentration distributions

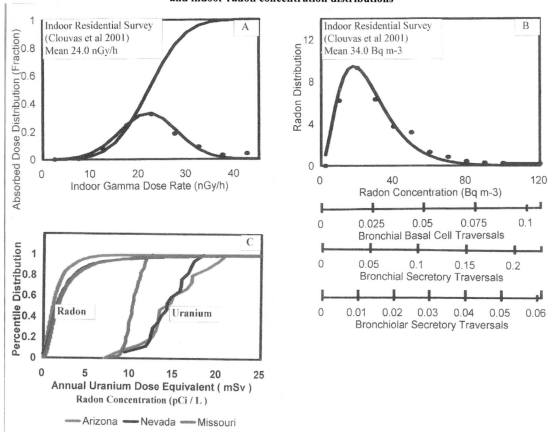

Figure 27 – Analysis of separate data by Clouvas et al (2001) showing indoor gamma ray dose rates and indoor radon concentration distributions. Also, comparisons of radon concentration (EPA) and terrestrial Uranium gamma ray dose (USGS), for Arizona, Nevada and Missouri, showing large variation in relative levels for the terrestrial Uranium gamma ray does depending on geological localities. Panel A – Clouvas gamma ray data. Panel B – Clouvas indoor radon data showing a Log-Normal Distribution. Panel C – Radon (EPA 2003) and Uranium gamma ray (USGS) data.

The distributions for the total indoor gamma ray dose rate is shown in Figure 27A and the distribution for the radon concentration is presented as Figure 27B. The gamma ray data reflects a Normal Distribution and the radon a Log-Normal Distribution. We show, for the radon data, the lung cell nucleus traversals for the three sensitive lung cell species based on James et al values given in our Figure 27B. Figure 27C shows the Percentile Distributions for Radon and Uranium Dose Equivalent showing a wide range. What is shown is that even on a local basis humans are exposed to a large range of radiation levels from the exposure sources, within the very large range of mean values worldwide. This means that one would expect to see a wide range of natural background and man-made radiation induced Adaptive Response radio-protection from the wide range of radon and progeny alpha induced lung damage as seen in the case-control studies (see Figure 2).

3.4 Correlation Between Terrestrial Uranium Gamma Ray Dose and Radon Indoor Concentration

It has been known that the Uranium series indoor gamma ray dose correlates with the indoor radon concentrations. This is because radon and its progeny are decay products in the Uranium series. Several investigators have examined this correlation. Clouvas et al (2003) performed a limited study comparing the Uranium series gamma dose rate with radon levels and found minimal correlation primarily due to a small number of data sets. Pilkyte and Butkus (2005) obtained measurements in 609 individual rooms in Lithuania and found considerable scatter in the data but a linear variation of Total Gamma Absorbed Dose Rate (nGy/h) = 121.5 nGy/h + 0.03 (nGy/h per Bq m^{-3}) C (Bq m^{-3}) where as noted C is radon indoor concentration in Bq m^{-3}.

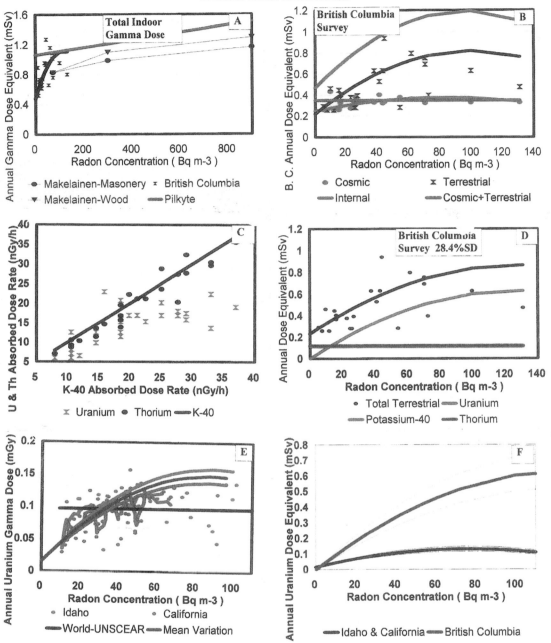

Figure 28 - Examination of correlation between variation in terrestrial Uranium gamma ray dose and variation in indoor radon concentration. Panel A – Graphical presentation of U gamma and radon data from Pilkyte et al (2005), Makelainen et al (2001) and the British Columbia radiation survey (BC 2008). Panal B – The variation of indoor cosmic ray, indoor terrestrial and internal dose with increasing indoor radon concentration. Panel C – A linear-quadratic least squares fit to the British Columbia terrestrial gamma ray dose.

We have converted the linear equation to Annual Gamma Dose in mSv (for gamma rays we let 1 mGy = 1 mSV for low LET radiations) and show the curve as a solid blue line in Figure 28A. Also, Makelainen et al (2001) examined a possible correlation in homes in Finland. They found a loose correlation and found a difference between wood and masonry constructed homes. Their three data points for each case (wood and masonry) are shown in Figure 28A. The most significant data on indoor gamma ray dose and radon concentration are that obtained by the Canadian province of British Columbia in a study of human indoor doses from natural and man-made radiations. The study was performed by the British Columbia Centre for Disease Control (BC 2008). From the data for 22 provincial territories, we provide, in Figure 28A, the terrestrial annual dose equivalent data is given by sorting with respect to radon concentration also in mSv. In Figure 28B, we show three of the components in the British Columbia study i.e. the cosmic ray gamma component which is found to vary slightly with increasing radon levels, the terrestrial gamma ray dose, the internal dose and the sum of the indoor gamma cosmic and terrestrial. The sum curve is the same as shown in Figure 28A. These data show that the terrestrial gamma ray dose increases with increasing indoor radon concentration. As we noted, it has been known that the Uranium content found in local soils and in building materials correlates with indoor radon concentration levels (as suggested by the Makelainen et al data and USGS). The connection with the Uranium series is because radon and its progeny are part of the Uranium decay series. A fundamental question is whether the Potassium-40 and Thorium series show some correlation also. Figure 28C provides a graph of the variation of U and Th, by ratios, with increasing observed K-40 levels. We see that the Th gamma ray dose is relatively linear with K-40 gamma ray dose. The Uranium dose shows significant variation indicating that the U dose varies with radon concentration where-as the other two gamma components are relatively constant. For the British Columbia data presented in Figure 28B, we can estimate the variation in Uranium with respect to indoor radon levels by assuming that UNSCEAR world-wide ratios for U, Th and K-40 are valid. From the Table I from the UNSCEAR (2000) report, the U, Th and K-40 values are 0.100, 0.160 and 0.150 mSv, respectively. By assuming that these relative values apply for BC at the median radon concentration of 24.3 Bq m^{-3} and the Th and K-40 dose equivalents remain constant at those levels, we obtain the variation in Uranium Dose Equivalent with radon concentration. We show this in Figure 28D.

In the previous section, we showed how, from location to location, the radiation levels vary considerably. Another estimation of the correlation between the Uranium series gamma terrestrial dose and radon concentration was obtained from the USGS Uranium Concentrations Data File by US counties from the High-Radon Project: (NURE 2008). The data is given in ppm Uranium. With the 5.48 nGy/h per U ppm conversion factor [see Equation (9)] the mean Uranium dose equivalent for each county is available. To accompany this data, we have used the EPA State Residential Radon Survey ASCII data (EPA 2008) which lists individual indoor radon measurements by county in each state. A total of over 51,000 data sets are provided. We have chosen the California and the Idaho state data sets and averaged the radon concentration results for each county in these two states. A total of 1886 indoor radon concentrations in the 53 counties were used for the California data. For Idaho, there were 1266 radon data sets for the 41 counties. Figure 28E provides the county averages data points as a function of radon concentration. Shown are also the separate 5 point smoothed curves, for California and Idaho, and the data least squares fitted to a linear-quadratic curve. The separate fits were very similar. For California, we obtained

Uranium Gamma Dose (mSv) = $0.014 + 0.0029\ C - 1.9 \times 10^{-5}\ C^2$ where C is radon concentration in Bq m^{-3}. For the Idaho data, we obtained

Uranium Gamma Dose (mSv) = $0.016 + 0.0032\ C - 2.1 \times 10^{-6}\ C^2$

The purple curve is the averaged composite fit with

Uranium Gamma Dose (mSv) = $0.015 + 0.00305\ C - 2.0 \times 10^{-6}\ C^2$ 　　(9)

For the over 3000 radon data sets, we find that there is a significant variation in Uranium gamma ray dose with increasing indoor radon levels. It is significant that, using the median radon concentration of 24.3 Bq m^{-3} in the Equation (9), we obtain a Uranium gamma dose of 0.0879 mSv per year. The UNSCEAR estimated world-wide value is 7 nGy/h = 0.0964 mSv per year for the low LET gamma rays. It is seen that, at very low radon levels, the Uranium gamma ray dose is about ½ the level at the mean radon concentration of 24.3 Bq m^{-3}. As Figure 28F, we provide the British Columbia and the composite CA and ID Uranium Gamma Ray Dose Equivalent curves with their estimated standard errors. We will use these estimates for the correlation of terrestrial Uranium gamma ray dose with indoor radon concentration and AR inducing charged particle traversals for the Uranium gammas with varying radon concentration.

3.5 Lung Dose from the Low LET Beta Rays Emitted from the Lung Deposited Radon Progeny

The radon gas and its progeny emit 14 different energy gamma rays and 7 different energy beta rays as seen in Figure A2. In most instances the effects of the radon progeny beta and gamma rays have been neglected when assessing the health risks from radon. This has been true for the BEIR Committee reports and even a recent extensive analysis by Kendall and Smith (2002) of doses to the lung and various other human organs and tissues. The neglect of these low LET radon progeny radiations is reasonably prudent since their LETs and hence RBEs are so much lower than the radon and progeny alpha particles as seen from the Miller et al (1995) data in Figure 8. The mean free path in tissue of the progeny gamma rays (Rockwell 1956) vary from about 5.6 cm (for the ^{222}Rn 0.19 MeV gamma ray) to about 22 cm (for the ^{214}Bi 2.44 MeV gamma), thus the gamma rays are correctly assumed to escape interaction to the lung tissue when emitted within the lung tissue itself from the deposited radon progeny. The case for the progeny betas is quite different in our effort to account for single traversals through the lung cells. As seen in the Figure 22, a progeny emitted beta ray is locally absorbed but traverses many cell diameters in its slowing down process. Only in a few cases involving radon research has radon progeny beta ray dose from radon progeny been evaluated, such as the extensive program of Cross et al (1988) *in vivo* exposure of dogs to high levels of radon and the *in vitro* exposure of human lymphocytes to radon progeny radiations (Pohl-Ruling 1988). A special team of dosimetry specialists evaluated the beta dose in the exposures (Jostes et al 1991) for both the Cross and Pohl-Ruling studies. For the Pohl-Ruling exposures they estimated that about 5% of the dose was radon progeny beta dose since radon gas was a principle exposure source as well as the progeny. This is because much of the betas energy is expended outside the very thin *in vitro* samples. For the beta rays emitted from the radon progeny deposited in the lung, we estimate the beta dose to be about 20% of the radon dose in mGy. The beta dose will vary linearly with radon concentration i.e. we let

$$\text{Beta Dose (in mGy)} = 0.20 \pm 0.05 \text{ x Radon Dose (in mGy)} \qquad (10)$$

Figure 29, Estimation of the variation in lung beta and uranium gamma ray dose

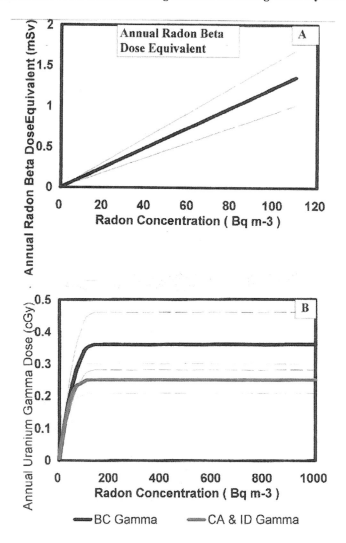

Figure 29 - Panel A – Estimation of the variation in lung beta dose from the radon progeny deposited in the lung as a function of radon concentration. Panel B – Estimation of the human lung dose from the terrestrial Uranium gamma ray dose as a function of radon concentration. Shown is the estimated based on the British Columbia and for the CA/ID data.

As Figure 29A, we show the radon progeny beta annual dose equivalent as a function of radon concentration. To consider the two lung radiation sources that are shown to vary with radon concentration (the U terrestrial shown in Figure 28D) and the radon betas, as Figure 29B we show the total variation of U terrestrial dose equivalent for the 30 day lung cells mitotic cycle from the British Columbia and the CA/ID data. Shown are the standard errors also.

4. ANALYSIS

4.1 Computation of the Lung Cells Specific Energy Hit Rate at UNSCEAR World-wide Average Low LET Human Exposure Rates

We have mentioned that, in Appendix A, we have computed the dose components for the UNSCEAR world-wide averages. We use a worldwide average radon concentration of 24.3 Bq m^{-3} for the Table A1 calculations. In Table A1, we provide the tabulation of the individual external and internal radiations making up the total exposures. Given are the energies of the betas and gamma rays, the percent of decays for each decay transition for K-40, the Uranium series, and the Thorium series.and the proton cosmic rays. Also given are the individual LETs for each radiation. In Table A1, the LETs for K-40 and the U and Th series are averaged based on their percentage of decays. From these the Specific Energy Depositions per Hit are computed and finally the Hits to the three sensitive lung cells for a 30 day mitotic cycle are given. In Table A2, we compute the mean Specific Energy Depositions per radiation induced charged particle through the three sensitive lung cell components, $<z_1>$. We provide the tabulation of the total charged particle traversals from all the components to examine the probability of single traversals to activate Adaptive Response protection. The Tables are described in more detail in Appendix A. From these calculations, we estimate that 0.338, 1.306 and 0.477 specific energy hits per cell cycle are received per basal, bronchial secretory and bronchiolar secretory cells, respectively, at the UNSCEAR world-wide average human annual radiation exposure levels given in Table 1. With these Poisson distributed mean Hits, 29%, 73% and 38% respectively of the three sensitive lung cells are protected. By neglecting the progeny beta dose and the Uranium gamma dose that vary with radon concentration, at zero radon concentration, 0.150, 0.656 and 0.239 cells are hit, providing about 10%, 58% and 20% Adaptive Response protection to humans not even exposed to radon.

4.2 Radon Variation - Combined Alpha Particle Bystander Effect and Adaptive Response Protection for UNSCEAR World-wide Average

We have concluded, for our evaluation here of the specific energy hits to the human lung cells, that an assumption of constant dose rates for the human doses from medical, cosmic, internal, Thorium series and Potassium-40, based on UNSCEAR world-wide averages is sufficient for our analysis. We have however concluded that the dose rates for the terrestrial Uranium series gamma rays and the beta ray dose rate from the deposited radon progeny must be treated as variable in our analysis. In Figure 29B, based on the terrestrial Uranium gamma ray dose variations with radon concentration from the British Columbia and the combination CA and ID data in Figure 28, we have provided the estimated variation in the doses from the terrestrial Uranium gamma ray dose in the two cases. Both are normalized to the UNSCEAR world average of 0.122 at the indoor radon median radon level of 24.3 Bq m^{-3}. We allow the Uranium dose to vary with radon level. We have then used the same method as in the Appendix A Tables A1 and A2 in Table A3 to compute the Specific Energy Hits per 30 day cycle as a function of varying radon concentration for the variation in beta dose with radon variation but for the two separate Uranium gamma ray variation cases.

Figure 30, British Columbia U gamma data. The variation in lung Specific Energy Hits for the separate dose components as a function of increasing radon concentration exposure

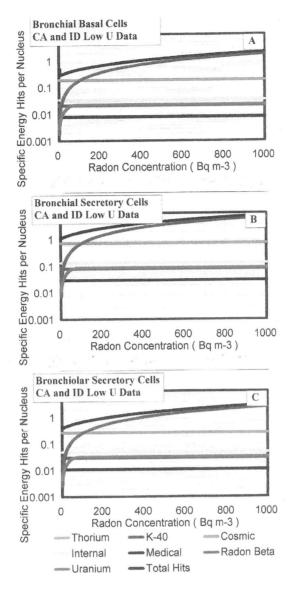

Figure 30 - British Columbia U gamma data. The variation in lung Specific Energy Hits for the separate dose components as a function of increasing radon concentration exposure. The cosmic, internal, medical external Thorium series and external K-40 are assumed constant at the UNSCEAR worldwide averages. The radon progeny beta and Uranium gamma doses are varied according to Figure 26 with increasing radon concentration. Panel A – Bronchial basal cells. Panel B – Bronchial secretory cells. Panel C – Bronchiolar secretory cells.

Figures 30A, 30B and 30C provide these data for the British Columbia for the three lung cell species.

Figure 31, Same as Figure 27 except for using the lower CA/ID U gamma ray data for Specific Energy Hits with increasing radon concentration

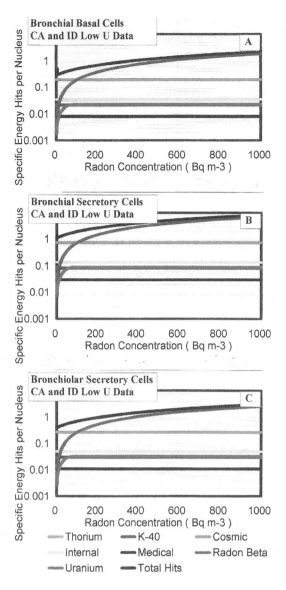

Figure 31 - Same as Figure 27 except for using the lower CA/ID U gamma ray data for Specific Energy Hits with increasing radon concentration.

Figures 31A, 31B and 31C provide the Specific Energy Hits per 30 day cycle for the CA/ID case. We show, in Table A3, each components contribution to the overall net Specific Energy Hits per Nucleus per 30 day cycle. Where the net Specific Energy Hits curve crosses unity, a Poisson mean of one charged particle traversal has occurred per cell nucleus.

Figure 32, British Columbia data and CA/ID data

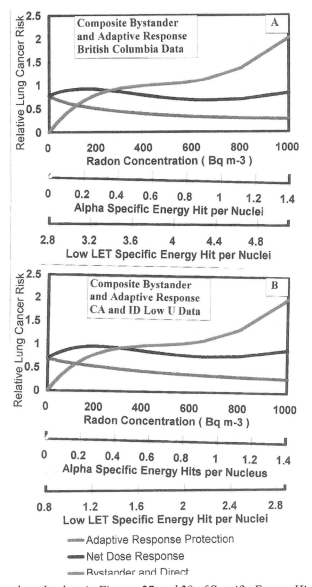

Figure 32 - Based on the data in Figures 27 and 28 of Specific Energy Hits, the estimated human lung dose response to alpha particle traversals (red curve) and to the Adaptive Response radio-protection (blue curve) and the combined effect on the human lung cancer risks with increasing radon concentration. Panel A – The British Columbia data from Figure 27. Panel B – the CA/ID data from Figure 28.

As Figures 32A and 32B we show the Adaptive Response protection factor in blue, the alpha particle Excess Relative Risk from the Bystander Effect and Direct Damage without AR protection and the Net Dose Response (in terms of Radon Lung Cancer Risk) considering the alpha particle damage and also the Adaptive Response protection against the damage from the Specific Energy Hits in Figures 30 and 31.

Having obtained an estimate of the variation in Adaptive Response radio-protection as a function of increasing radon concentration at the residential radon level up to 1000 Bq m^{-3}, we now can estimate the reduction in Relative Lung Cancer Risk starting with the dose response curves in Figure 16. Figure 16C extends the radon level to 2500 Bq m-3. In Figure 32 herein, for the UNSCEAR world-wide average doses, still comparing the British Columbia and the CA/ID separate calculations, we show this normalized representative alpha particle dose response, without AR reduction (red curve), from Figure 16. The blue curve is the magnitude of the AR protection based on the estimate in Figure 30 of Specific Energy Hits (next to last column in Table A3) and the Table A3 calculation of AR protection (last column). The black curve is the net Relative Lung Cancer Risk for the two calculations (BC and CA/ID). We see that there is little difference in the results in separately considering the estimated terrestrial Uranium gamma ray dose based on the British Columbia data and the California and Idaho (CA/ID) data. In the subsequent analysis, in Figures 33 and 34, we will report the use of only the British Columbia data known to be more accurate since they were field measured.

4.3 Examination of the Radon Relative Risks for the UNSCEAR Maximum and Minimum Variations in Human Low LET Radiations to Humans

Examining the EPA High-Radon Project data, the USGS Terrestrial Gamma Ray data, the California Gamma Ray data of Woolenberg et al (1994), the residential data of Clouvas et al (2001) and other data presented here in Sections 3.2.c and 3.2.d, we have shown that there is a very large variation in the human radiation exposures based on geographic location worldwide. For this reason, from the Table 1 UNSCEAR typical range of human radiation exposures by component, we have performed calculations for the low range values and the high range values of annual exposures. In the low range case we used – cosmic rays 0.30 mSv; Terrestrial gamma 0.30 mSv (U gamma 0.073 mSv; Th gamma 0.117 mSv; K-40 gamma 0.110 mSv); internal 0.20 mSv; and medical 0.02 mSv.

Figure 33, the range of Adaptive Response radio-protection

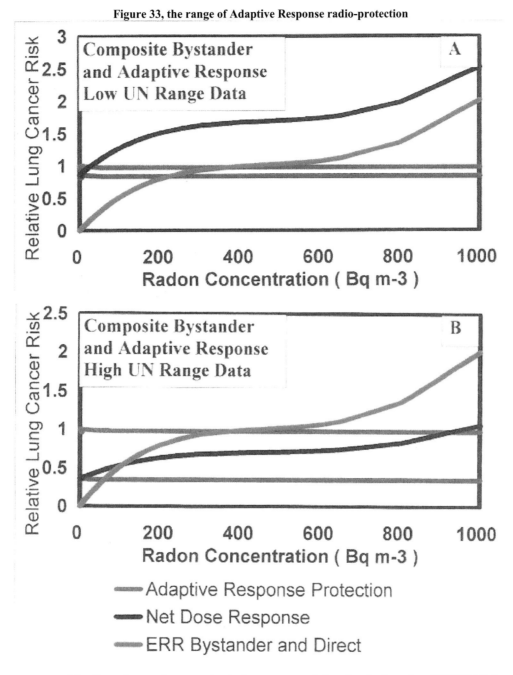

Figure 33 - Considering the variation in human annual dose levels, based on UNSCEAR data, from variation in geological and ecological conditions, the estimated maximums and minimums are used to calculate the range of Adaptive Response radio-protection that may be expected from the range of Specific Energy Hits based on these variations. Panel A – Maximum for British Columbia Uranium dose data. Panel B – Maximum for CA/ID data. Panel C – Minimum for British Columbia data. Panel D – Minimum for CA/ID data.

Figure 33A provides the Radon Relative Risks for the UNSCEAR low range human exposure values. As Figure 33B, we show the maximum range calculations (High human low LET radiation exposures.). Here we used - cosmic rays 1.00 mSv; Terrestrial gamma 0.60 mSv (U gamma 0.146 mSv; Th gamma 0.234 mSv; K-40 gamma 0.220 mSv); internal 0.80 mSv; and medical 1.20 mSv. These large variations support a large variation in human lung cancer risks for the case-control studies shown in Figures 2A and 2B for the case-control studies, which are further studied in Chapter 4 - Part III. The normalized alpha particle representative dose response given in Figure 16 further supports a non-linear BaD Model type dose response in the large variations in Figures 32 and 33. This will be shown to be true, in Chapter 4 - Part III, for the case-control studies. There is a difference relative to the expected dose response from case-control studies and what we have predicted in Figures 32 and 33 for combined Bystander and Adaptive Response effects. Since case-control studies involve comparisons between lung cancer and non-lung cancer cohorts in the same geological and ecological settings they are normalized to unity at zero radon exposure and not worldwide or national "spontaneous" lung cancer rates (without radon exposure). We show this normalization of the Appendix A calculations to unity for case-control studies in Figure 34.

Figure 34, Normalization of British Columbia Data to Controls

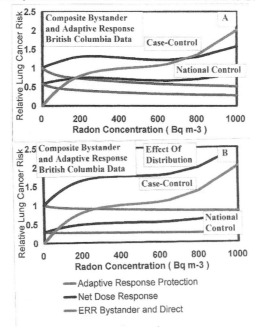

Figure 34 – For the British Columbia data in Figure 32A, we show the effect of normalization to controls at zero radon concentration with, in Panel A, the upper Adaptive Response protection (in blue) and normalized case-control Net Dose Response (in black). Panel B is estimate of normalized case-control with a distribution of background levels.

5. SUMMARY

In Part I of this three part study, alpha particle and other high LET broad-beam and micro-beam *in vitro* data (Miller et al 1976, 1995, 1999, Zhou et al 2001, 2004, Nagasawa and Little 1999, 2002, Hei et al 1999, Sawant et al 2001) were examined with the Brenner et al (2001) microdosimetry, Bystander BaD Model. This model has been used by others (Little and Wakeford 2001, Little 2004, Brenner and Sachs 2002, 2003, Brenner 1994, Brenner et at 2001) with the *a priori* assumption that at least some radon induced human lung cancers are caused by Bystander damaged cells. It was found that for alpha particles with LETs near that of radon progeny alpha particles, that a standard Representative Alpha Particle Dose Response shape with BaD Model parameters within ± 10% SD when scaled to microdose alpha particle cell traversals. This standard representative shape was then normalized to the BEIR VI (1999) Relative Risk at 400 Bq m-3 radon concentration to provide a best estimate of human lung cancer Relative Risk dose response. This best estimate is non-linear with the lung cancer incidence at low radon domestic levels from Bystander cellular damage and at high underground miner radon levels from direct alpha traversals.

This Part II here, of the three part study, has examined the potential influence of the Adaptive Response radio-protection on human lung cancer risks from radon. The radiation source of this protection is considered to be the natural background and man-made radiation to which humans are exposed on a day-to-day bases. The UNSCEAR (2001) world-wide estimate of human radiation exposures, Table I, is used for the radiation source components. Fundamental to the examination process is the knowledge that single low LET charged particle traversals activates the AR protective mechanism, it persists for at least one mitotic cell cycle, is relatively independent of the inducing low LET radiations and produces a reduction in both radiation induced and natural spontaneous chromosome damage by 50 to 80% (Leonard 2005, 2007a, 2007b, 2008a, 2008b, 2008c).

It is shown from a number of radiation surveys that there is a very wide range of natural background and man-made exposures from region-to-region and even in localized areas within regions. The Appendix A, Tables A1, A2 and A3 computes the Specific Energy Hits and Adaptive Response protection factors to the three carcinogenically sensitive lung cell species at the UNSCEAR world-wide average (40% AR reduction), with the estimated variation radon level and with the maximum (80% AR reduction) and

101

minimum (20% AR reduction) range of human low LET exposures. Each Relative Risk curve (Figures 32, 33 and 34) show non-linear Bystander Damage dose response for residential and workplace human exposures and Direct Damage for underground miner exposures.

Chapter 4 - PART III - EVIDENCE OF INFLUENCE OF COMBINED BYSTANDER AND ADAPTIVE RESPONSE EFFECTS ON RADON CASE-CONTROL STUDIES

1. INTRODUCTION

1.1 Microdose Analysis of Case-Control Studies

Radon lung cancer studies have been performed using the case-control method of data collection and analysis. BEIR VI (1999) provides lung cancer risk data from some of the early case-control studies in their Figure 3-2. These studies involve the matching of each human lung cancer case with one or more non-cancer cohorts with similar demographic characteristics. In these studies, both cases and controls are matched with exposures to similar levels of low Radon concentrations. Such studies have been performed in Europe (13 studies) and North America (8 studies) with these data recently being pooled by several analysis groups to provide more statistical power (Darby et al 2005, 2006, Krewski et al 2005, 2006). We show the linearized fit of the studies as Figure 2. Table 3 here provides the Odds Ratio data for the Krewski studies. At the request of the Darby group we only show their Figure 2A graphs.

Table 3 Adjusted Odds Ratios (SE) and Corresponding 95% Confidence Intervals as a Function of Radon Exposure Categories for Eight Sites in North America. Values in brackets are 95%CLs

Study	<25	25 -- <50	50 -- <75	75 -- <100	100 -- <150	150 -- <199	≥ 200
CT	1.00	1.15 (0.26) [0.73, 1.79]	1.27 (0.41) [0.67, 2.39]	0.78 (0.36) [0.31, 1.94]		1.37 (0.50) [0.66, 2.81]	
IA	1.00		2.10 (0.72) [1.07, 4.11]	1.68 (0.60) [0.84, 3.38]	2.02 (0.68) [1.04, 3.92]	2.43 (0.87) [1.21, 4.89]	1.90 (0.65) [0.97, 3.72]
MA	1.00	0.53 (0.21) [0.24, 1.13]	0.31 (0.14) [0.13, 0.73]		0.47 (0.20)[a] [0.20, 1.10]	0.22 (0.18)[b] [0.04, 1.13]	2.50 (2.15)[c] [0.47, 13.46]
MO-I	1.00	1.01 (0.27) [0.59, 1.72]	1.00 (0.29) [0.57, 1.75]	0.99 (0.34) [0.51, 1.92]		1.35 (0.43) [0.72, 2.52]	
MO-IIa	1.00	0.43 (0.18) [0.19, 0.98]	1.02 (0.48) [0.41, 2.57]	0.71 (0.37) [0.25, 1.98]		0.57 (0.29) [0.21, 1.54]	
MO-IIg	1.00	1.03 (0.35) [0.45, 2.01]	1.07 (0.33) [0.51, 1.97]	1.03 (0.38) [0.54, 2.12]		1.56 (0.59) [0.68, 3.26]	
NJ	1.00	0.82 (0.24) [0.47, 1.46]	1.10 (0.65) [0.34, 3.51]	0.65 (0.83) [0.05, 7.87]	0.27 (0.26) [0.04, 1.84]		
UT-ID	1.00	1.00 (0.31) [0.55, 1.84]	1.58 (0.56) [0.79, 3.15]	1.62 (0.68) [0.71, 3.70]		1.44 (0.57) [0.67, 3.11]	
Winn	1.00		1.03 (0.61) [0.33, 3.27]	1.78 (0.99) [0.60, 5.27]	0.77 (0.39) [0.29, 2.06]	1.90 (1.20) [0.55, 6.56]	1.13 (0.60) [0.40, 3.21]

[a] OR for 75 - <150 Bq m^{-3}.
[b] OR for 150 - < 200 Bq m^{-3}.
[c] OR for ≥ 250 Bq m^{-3}.

The pooling of data from these studies is based on the assumption "that between-site differences seen in the observed relationship between lung cancer risk and radon exposure are due to random measurement variability and the true relationship is independent of site locality and only dependent on the carcinogenic sensitivity of human lung tissue to alpha radiation", which both Darby et al (2005, 2006) assumed to be Linear No-Threshold (LNT) compatible with BEIR VI (1999). BEIR VI (1999) summarized their justification of LNT for human lung cancer risk as follows: "The choice was to use a linear relationship between risk and low doses of radon progeny without a threshold. The choice was based primarily on considerations related to the stochastic nature of the energy deposition by alpha particles; at low doses, a decrease in dose simply results in a decrease in the number of cells subjected to the same insult. That observation, combined with the evidence that a single alpha particle can cause substantial permanent damage to a cell and that most cancers are of monoclonal origin, provides the mechanistic basis of the use of a linear model at low doses. In addition, as discussed in the report, exposure-response relationships estimated from the observational data in miners with low exposures, and from the case-control studies of indoor radon, are consistent with linearity."

Of considerable significance is the very recent case-control lung cancer epidemiological study of Thompson et al (2008), for Worcester County, Massachusetts (making now a total of 9 North America studies), showing a significant reduction of lung cancer incidence with increasing residential Radon concentrations. Since the BEIR VI (1999) was issued, a large amount of new research data has been published about low level radiation dose response, primarily sponsored by the United States Department of Energy Low Radiation Dose Research Program. We here report Part III of a three part study of the combined influence from the deleterious behavior of the Bystander Effect (BE) and from the radio-protective behavior of Adaptive Response (AR), on the human health risks from radon. In the separate Chapter 2 - Part I of this study, we have shown that cellular dose response from radon progeny and other similar high LET alpha particles, in the absence of any low LET radiation inducing AR, can be typified by a Representative Alpha Particle Dose Response shape and accurately characterized by a modified microdose BaD Bystander Model (with some minor modifications given in Chapter 2 - Part I) first proposed by Brenner et al (2001). It is shown, for radon concentrations at human domestic and workplace levels, as provided by the BEIR VI (1999) report, that the carcinogen causing cellular chromosome damage in the human lung must be from Bystander Damage to neighboring cells adjacent to directly hit cells. This is based on the latest evaluation of the human lung cells alpha particle "hit" (traversal) rate per Bq m^{-3} of radon exposure provided by James et al (2004). The Bystander Damage dose response, from broad-beam and micro-beam *in vitro* data, is shown to be non-monotonic concave downward in shape for human domestic level, low radon exposures. Only at the higher radon levels received by the underground miners would the dose response be from cellular/alpha particle Direct Damage and linear or linear-quadratic as provided by many other published alpha dose response data. This representative dose response shape is provided in Part I as Figure 10 (Leonard et al 2010a) and the explicit shapes in the low radon residential Bystander region is given in

105

Figure 16B. It is concluded that the dose response for lung cancer risks from radon should not be expected to be Linear No-Threshold, contrary to Figure 3-2 of BEIR VI (1999) (see the bottom panel of Figure 1, Part I), and contrary to the pooled linear fits to the European and North American case-control data analysis shown in Figure 2 of Part I. The basic evidence presented in Part I, from *in vitro* data, is that the Bystander Effect from radon and progeny alpha particles is dominant in inducing lung cancer in humans from radon at residential levels.

Conversely in the separate Chapter 3 - Part II, we examined the potential influence of combined deleterious Bystander Effect and Adaptive Response radio-protection by assuming, based also on a very large amount of *in vitro* BE and AR data, that AR is operable for low LET ionizing radiations that humans routinely receive from natural background and man-made radiations. Significant to the Part II study of potential Adaptive Response effects on the human lung cancer risks from radon is the fact that single low LET radiation induced charged particle tracks through sensitive regions of cells induces an AR protection of 40 to 70 % against chromosome damage. This has been evidenced after the Poisson threshold transition region of AR dose response data such as that of Azzam et al (1996) and Redpath et al (2001, 2003) [see Figures 2A and 2B of Leonard (2007a)]. Further, Sawant et al (2001) and Zhou et al (2003) have shown that low LET X-ray priming doses can reduce the transformation frequency rate and level of chromosome aberrations from alpha particle exposures (see Figures 19A and 19B) . The Adaptive Response protection is found to be independent of the type of radiations, from 28 keV mammogram X-rays to 232 Mev cosmic ray protons, and independent of cell species for five different cell species although the level of protection and the dose range of the protection does vary somewhat dependent on the specific energy deposition of the single low LET charged particle traversals (see Figure 21). In examining whether Adaptive Response may induce radio-protection against the alpha particle induced human lung damage, we used the United Nations Scientific Committee on the Effects of Atomic Radiations (UNSCEAR 2000) estimated human exposures to ionizing radiations as the AR inducing radiation sources. It was found, at the world-wide mean radiation levels, that about 30% of the human lung cells should experience AR radio-protection and at the high UNSCEAR (2000) levels 100% of human lung cells should receive AR protection. From Chapter 2 - Part I and Chapter 3 – Part II, we show that the human lung cancer risk dose response should be non-linear from alpha particle cell damage and further, different

106

ecological and geographical environments world-wide should impose a large range Adaptive Response radio-protection and a wide range of observed odds ratios of lung cancer risk as is indeed observed in the European (13 studies) and North American (8 studies) case-control studies as seen in Figure 2. This is supportive of the non-linear premises of Morgan (2006). Based on these premises, in this Chapter 4 - Part III, we examine the odds ratio data for these 21 pooled studies, the very recent Massachusetts study of Thompson et al (2008) and the China study of Blot et al (1990) for non-linear lung cancer risks as expected from the results of Chapter 2 - Part I and Chapter 3 – Part II.

2. MATERIALS AND METHODS

2.1 Method - Recent Case-Control Studies May Provide Insight Into the Variation of Bystander Damage and Adaptive Response Radio-Protection From Human Lung Cancer

We provide as Figure 2 of Part I the reproduction of the graphs of data and their linearized fits for the Darby et al (2005, 2006) pooled 13 European case-control and the Krewski et al (2005, 2006) pooled 8 North American case-control studies. It was most likely a large disappointment for the participants in the pooled studies to find such a very large variation in the Odds Ratio Relative Lung Cancer Risks as a function of increasing radon concentration for the different geographical localities. In the Results Section herein, we analyze these 21 data sets plus the Shengyang, China (Blot et al 1990) study and the very recent Massachusetts (MA) (Thompson et al 2008) study. We first examine the validity of the assumption of linearity that was assumed to produce Figure 2 of Part I, where a very wide range in linearized slopes is observed for both the Krewski et al (2005, 2006) and Darby et al (2005, 2006) pooled data with some showing negative lung cancer risks with increasing radon levels. Due to this wide range, we then divided the data into two groups, i.e. positive sloped (high risk group) and negative sloped (low risk group) sets, and performed single linear fits. Because our Part I and II analysis concludes that radon lung cancer risks should not be expected to be Linear No-Threshold, we next considered, without imposing explicitly any Adaptive Response criteria, that there may be more than the Linear No-Threshold mechanisms affecting the dose responses. The well known Papworth Poisson Validation Test (Papworth 1975, Savage and Papworth 2000) was applied and revealed that a single linear mechanism premise to be invalid, showing over-dispersion of the data for a hypothesis of a single linear cancer risk mechanism as premised in BEIR VI (1999). To examine a hypothesis, premised from the Part I and II results, that BE and AR influence should produce non-linear human lung cancer risk behavior, both the Darby et al (2005, 2006) plus China (Blot et al 1990) and the Krewski et al (2005, 2006) plus MA (Thompson et al 2008) data low risk group and the high risk group sets were each trial fit to 3rd, 4th and 5th degree polynomials. With the suspect that they may reflect minimal radon induced lung cancer response, the three lowest risk data sets of the Krewski et al (2005, 2006) plus Massachusetts (MA) data sets, i.e. the Massachusetts (MA). New Jersey (NJ) and Missouri (MO-IIa) data in Table 1, were then individually fit to the basic Microdose Model for Adaptive Response protection (Leonard 2007a), given as Equation (3) of Part II, i.e. neglecting any Bystander lung damage, with excellent success. These three lung cancer risk sets thus show a net AR protection against lung cancer with increasing radon levels which significantly reflects also a reduction in naturally occurring, spontaneous lung cancers from non-radon causes by being below the zero radon cancer incident rates.

In Chapter 6, we discuss the validity of *in vitro* data to predict *in vivo* human dose response and provide recent *in vivo* data of live mammalian examples of Adaptive Response protection.

3. RESULTS

3.1 Linear Analysis of Krewski et al (2005, 2006) and Darby et al (2005, 2006) Case-Control Data

Table 3 provides the numerical values for the odds ratios of lung cancer risks for the radon concentrations reported by Krewski et al (2005, 2006) and MA (Thompson et al 2008) studies. At the request of the Darby et al (2005, 2006) group, we only provide their graphical presentation in Figure 2A but used their numerical data in our analysis herein. What is very apparent, from the Figure 2A from Darby et al (2005, 2006) and Figure 2B from Krewski et al (2005, 2006), is that there is a very large variation in the linearized odds ratios slopes in lung cancer risks from the respective 13 different European and 9 different geographical locations in North America. In particular, the behavior of the 2 data sets, from New Jersey – NJ (Schoenberg et al 1990, 1992) and Missouri – MO-IIa (Alavanja et al 1994, 1999), show very clearly a strongly non-conforming negative behavior. The odds ratios in the Thompson et al (2008) MA data shown in their Figure 2 compliments the NJ and MO-IIa negative risk results for radon exposure values below about 200 Bq m^{-3}. The extreme differences suggests that more than one dose response mechanism may be present in the induction, and other cases of lack of induction, of radon induced lung cancer in humans, contrary to BEIR VI (1999) and Krewski et al (2005, 2006) and Darby (2005, 2006) premises.

First it is appropriate to more carefully assess the likelihood that the 9 North America lung cancer risk data in Table 3 represent a linear cancer induction mechanism as premised by the Linear No-Threshold hypothesis and shown in Figure 3-2 of BEIR VI (1999) and the bottom panel of Figure 1, Part I. The BEIR VI (1999) lung cancer Relative Risk is given by Equation (1), Section 3 of BEIR VI (1999) i.e.

$$\text{Relative Risk } (RR) = 1 + \beta w \qquad (1)$$

where w is the radon exposure and β estimates the increment in excess relative risk (ERR) for unit change in exposure. For their Figure 3-2, a value of about $\beta = 0.0019$ per Bq m^{-3} is used. Table 3 provides the odds ratio, standard error and 95%CL data values reported from Krewski et al (2005, 2006) and the values from Thompson et al (2008).

Figure 35, Linear best fit of Krewski plus MA and Darby plus China data

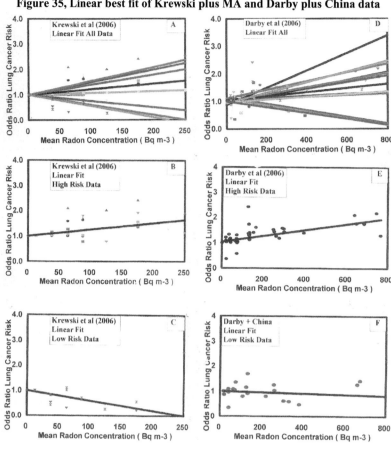

Figure 35 - Linear best fit of Krewski plus MA and Darby plus China data. Panel A - Use of the Method of Maximum Likelihood (MLE) to obtain a linear best fit to each of the eight North American lung cancer case-control studies pooled by Krewski et al (2005, 2006) and the Thompson et al (2008) case-control study for Worcester County, Massachusetts. Panel B – Use of MML to fit the high risk pooled group, i.e. CT, IA, UT-ID, MO-I, MO-IIg and Winn, to linear best fit. Panel C – Use of MML to fit the low risk North American pooled group i.e. NJ, MA and MO-IIa to linear best fit. Panel D – The MML linear best fit of each data set of the Darby and China 14 data sets. Panel E - Use of MML to fit the Darby high risk pooled group, to a linear best fit. Panel F - Use of MML to fit the low risk Darby and China pooled group i.e. United Kingdom, Spain, Western Germany and China to linear best fit.

As Figure 35A, we show our linearized best fit, obtained using the Method of Maximum Likelihood Estimation (Savage and Papworth 2000), for each of the 8 Krewski et al (2005, 2006) North American case-control studies and the new MA data of Thompson et al (2008) i.e. the data in Table 3. We see an extreme variation in the linear slopes for the individual sets when premised by the Linear No-Threshold (LNT) hypothesis. We obtained a range of values of β's from -0.0043 per Bq m^{-3} for NJ to +0.0049 per Bq m^{-3} for Iowa (IA). It does not seem plausible, if the data indeed reflects the lung cancer incidence rate from radon, that there would be negative risk with increasing radon concentration, if indeed world-wide the true lung cancer risk is given by a single value of β. We have next separated the Krewski et al (2005. 2006) data sets into two groups, one group including all the positive sloped, high risk data sets i.e. CT, IA, M)-I, MO-IIg, UT-ID and Winn. The second low risk group includes the three negative responding sets i.e. the MA, MO-IIa and the NJ sets. We have pooled each group and provide the high risk group linear fit as Figure 35B and the linear fit for the low risk group as Figure 35C.

The Darby et al (2005, 2006) pooled data have also been examined in the same way. As Figure 35D, we provide the linearized fit to each of the 13 European data sets and the China data set. Again we find a very large range for the Excess Relative Risk slopes. We again divided the Darby et al (2005, 2006) data into a positive sloped, high risk group (Austria, France, Czech Republic, Eastern Germany, Sweden Nationwide, Sweden never-smokers, Sweden Stockholm, Southern Finland and Italy). The low risk group, containing the negative responding and negligible risk results of Spain, United Kingdom, Western Germany, Finland Nationwide and China. As Figures 35E and 35F, we show the pooled linear fits to these two groups.

3.2 Statistical Considerations Relative to the Excessive Odds Ratios – A Poisson Fit Test

We have cited in the Introduction section the BEIR VI (1999) summary statement premising linearity of lung cancer risks from radon. Both the Krewski et al (2005, 2006) and the Darby et al (2005, 2006) studies are premised that "The pooling of data from these studies is based on the assumption that between-site differences seen in the observed relationship between lung cancer risk and radon exposure are due to random measurement variability and the true relationship is independent of site locality and only dependent on the carcinogenic sensitivity of human lung tissue to alpha radiation." These two pooled studies encompass a very large amount of case-control data. The following are the case and control data values for the noted case/control studies; Krewski et al (2005, 2006) 4081 and 5281 persons, Darby et al (2005, 2006) 7148 and 14208 persons, Thompson et al (2008) 209 and 397 persons, Shenyang, China (Blot et al 1990) 308 and 356 persons comprising a total of 11746 cases and 20242 controls. Analysis of the net population and of the two separate groups i.e. North America including MA data and the European plus China data for linearity should provide a reasonable estimate of the "true" linear slope constant, β, in Equation (1) for human lung cancer risk versus radon exposure concentration. Thus for each radon concentration data point, the deviation from the linearized risk curve should be from "radon measurement variability" (thus Poisson distribution) and, due to the large populations in the studies, the linearized risk curve should represent the "true relationship (which) is independent of site locality". Thus, a "universal" lung cancer risk. if it exists? The fits clearly show a very large variation in the lung cancer incidence rates from the various geographical locations in North America, Europe and China. Our evaluation, from odds ratio studies shown in Figure 35, is that a statistically significant difference in the slopes between the sites with a positive Excess Odds Ratios (EOR) and the sites with negative EOR provides evidence to reject, as a null hypothesis, the premise that the EOR's obtained from all the sites estimate one underlying single linear association between lung cancer risk and radon concentrations. We statistically evaluate the hypothesis.

Papworth (1975) was one of the first to observe that, if experimental data represented a physical process containing a mean value, then the distribution of data about the mean value should be Poisson distributed about this mean value if the data variations are related to only random variations in data collection and assessment i.e. in the case here, radon data taking processes in obtaining the case-control values. A Poisson Validation Test is standard procedure in evaluating the validity of chromosome assay data in radiation biology. The Cytogenetic Analysis for radiation dose assessment applies the Poisson Validation Test in the data analysis related to human overexposures in accident situations (IAEA 2001). For each dose data point on the dose response calibration, thousands of cells are scored for chromosome aberration frequency at each calibration dose data point. The distribution of these scored values about the mean value are tested for Poisson conformity. If the variance to mean ratio is large the data are considered to be over-dispersed.

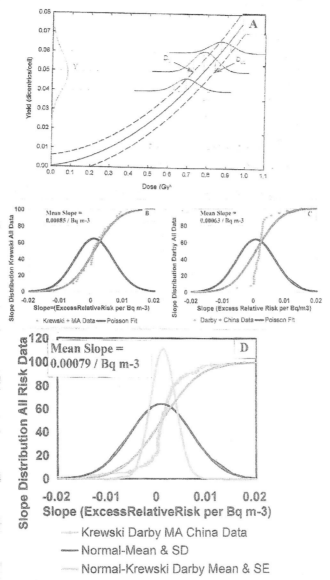

Figure 36 - Statistical evaluation of the case-control data sets for validity of the data. Panel A – Schematic illustration of the data distribution about individual data points in a chromosome aberration dose response curve, where each data point is a result of scoring a large number of cells, exposed to the same dose, for aberrations to obtain a statistical Mean Value for that dose point. The aberration distribution from the scoring is tested (Papworth Poisson Validation Test) for validity by fitting to a Poisson Distribution about the Mean Value. Panel B – The frequency distribution of the slopes of the Krewski plus MA data and fit to a Normal Distribution, showing the very large variation about the Mean Value of 0.00085 per Bq m-3. Panel C – The frequency distribution of the slopes of the Darby plus China data and fit to a Normal Distribution with a Mean Value of 0.00063 per Bq m-3. Panel D – The frequency distributions of the slopes of all the individual data from all the 23 case-control studies encompassing 109 data points of Odds Ratio Lung Cancer Relative Risks. The Mean Value is 0.00079 per Bq m-3.

Figure 36A illustrates the distribution behavior about the data points on a cytogenetic dose response calibration curve, reproduced from Figure 3 of Szluinska et al (2005). For the Excessive Odds Ratio Lung Cancer Risk data, if the cancer risk rate is indeed linear and independent of any other mechanisms other than Linear No-Threshold dose response for radon human lung cancer risks, then the best fit slope [value of β in Equation (1)] predicted by each radon concentration dose point on the dose response curve should be an assessment of the true linear curve. So for each case-control data point in each data set i.e. Spain, United Kingdom, France, etc. an experimental estimated value for the true slope is provided by the relation

$$\beta_{exp} = \text{Experimental Excess Odds Ratio / Mean Radon Concentration (w)} \qquad (2)$$

Then pooling the case-control data sets should provide a number of independent Slope Estimates. If Lung Cancer Risk is indeed independent of geographical location, as must have been premised by the participants in the two pooled studies, then the experimental β_{exp} values must form a Poisson distribution about the true linear slope value, β, for human lung cancer risk from radon. We have used the computer "U-Test for Poisson" program of the Poisson Test system "CTAMPOISS" from the United Kingdom Health Protection Agency (HPA 2008). We show the results in Figures 36B and 36C. We have graphically examined the frequency distribution of the Slope Estimate data points given by Equation (2). Figure 36B provides the distribution of the Equation (2) slope values for all the Krewski (2005, 2006) plus the Thompson et al (2008) MA data. The mean value of the slopes is 0.00085 per Bq m^{-3} of radon with a very large standard error (SE) of 0.00616. This is a lower slope than the 0.0011 per Bq m^{-3} value obtained by Krewski et al (2005, 2006) but we have included the Thompson et al (2008) MA negatively responding data. Similarly, shown in Figure 36C, we performed the same analysis for the Darby et al (2005, 2006) plus China (Blot et al 1990) data, again obtaining a lower slope value equal to 0.00063 per Bq m^{-3} slope value due to the China data, with a large SE of 0.00629, compared to 0.0011 for the Darby et al (2005, 2006) data. The CTAMPOISS Poisson Validation Test concludes that both the Krewski et al (2005, 2006) and Darby et al (2005, 2006) slope data set distributions are over-dispersed and were, on a technical basis, statistically rejected as being from a single mechanism and are "contaminated" from outlier influence. The very large standard errors are indicative of this Poisson Test failure. We performed a similar test of the entire pooled data of Krewski et al (2005, 2006), Darby et al (2005, 2006), MA (Thompson et al 2008) and China (Blot et al 1990). This is presented as Figure 36D showing a Mean Value of 0.00079 per Bq m-3 with a large SE of 0.00617. The spread of the Normal distribution is due to the large negative and positive slope values about the overall mean as shown by the data. In all the slope analysis the standard errors were 7 to 10 times larger than the Mean Slopes, supporting the overall purely statistical conclusion, provided by the Papworth (1975) Poisson Tests, that 1.) a simple linear fit to all the pooled data sets is inadequate and the *a priori* assumption of LNT cannot yield a reasonable, single linear dose response between lung cancer risk and radon exposure at domestic and workplace levels 2.) there are other mechanisms affecting the Human Lung Cancer Risks as determined by the case-control studies. We also used a second, more recent, Poisson Validation program, NETA also based on Edwards et al (1979), available through the Inter-net and obtained the same results and conclusions.

3.3 The Fit of the Krewski et al (2005, 2006) and the Darby et al (2005, 2006) Case-Control Lung Cancer Studies Data to Polynomials

Allowing for non-linearity, without a presumption that it be from Adaptive Response radio-protection, we have then used MML to trial fits of all the data sets to 3rd, 4th and 5th degree polynomials, $a + bX + cX^2 + dX^3 + eX^4 + fX^5$, which thus allows for considerable non-linearity if the data so dictates.We have fit the Darby et al (2005, 2006) data plus China (Blot et al 1990) data to these polynomials.

Figure 37, Two pooled data sets, from Table 3 and Figure 2 of part 1, fit to polynomials using the Method of Maximum Likelihood

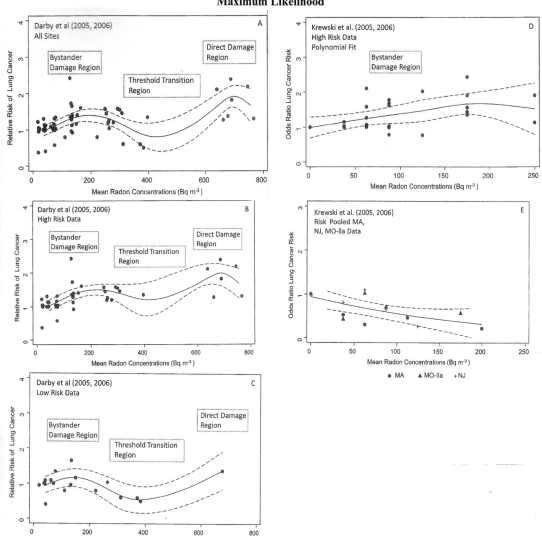

Figure 37 - Two pooled data sets, from Table 3 and Figure 2 of part 1, fit to polynomials using the Method of Maximum Likelihood. Panel A – Fit of 5th degree polynomial to all of the Darby et al (2005, 2006) and China case-control data. Panel B – The positive, high risks case-control data sets (Austria, France, Czech Republic, Eastern Germany, Sweden nationwide, Sweden Stockholm, Sweden never-smokers, Southern Finland and Italy) fit to 4th degree polynomials. Panel C – The pooled data fit for the low risk Darby data sets (United Kingdom, Western Germany, Spain, Finland nationwide and China) to 3rd degree polynomials. Panel D – The North American positive, high risks case-control data sets (CT, MO-I, MO-IIg, IA, UT-ID and Winn) fit to 4th degree polynomials. Panel E – The pooled data fit for the low risk North American data sets (MA, NJ and MO-IIa) to 3rd degree polynomials.

The best fits to the data sets are shown in Figure 37 with the 95% confidence limits. For the high risk data set, a 5th degree polynomial gave the best results with the polynomial coefficients: a = 0.93, b = 4.84 E-04, c = 4.87 E-05, d= -2.74 E-07, e= 5.03 E-10, and f = -2.97E-13, with an adjusted R^2 = 0.420. These are shown as Figure 4A, for

116

the high risk group. In Figure 4B, for the low risk group, we found a 5th degree polynomial provided the best fit with a = 0.836, b = 1.07 E-03, c = 4.85 E-05. e = 9.23 E-10 and f= -6.56 E-13, with an adjusted R^2 = 0.254. For the overall Darby et al (2005, 2006) data, we find a = 0.94, b = -9.28 E-04, c = 6.59 E-05, d = -3.67 E-07, e = 6.72 E-10, and f = -3.94 E-13 with an adjusted R^2 = 0.392. We see a significant resemblance to the Representative alpha Particle Dose Response data presented and analyzed in Chapter 2 - Part I and low radon concentration region of the Representative Alpha Particle Dose Response shape in Figure 10. We analyze this in more detail in Section 4.1.

For both the high and low risk group Krewski et al (2005, 2006) plus MA (Thompson et al 2008) polynomial fits, we found that a 2nd degree polynomial provided the best fit because their data only goes to about 300 Bq m^{-3}.(i.e. >200) in Table 3. As Figure 4C, we show the pooled CT, UT-ID, MO-I, MO-IIg, Winn and IA positive sloped high risk data sets, with the polynomial coefficients a = 0.987, b = 4.14 E-03, c = 9.51 E-05, d = -2.15 E-07, e = 1.22 E-09, and f = -2.02 E-12, with an adjusted R^2 = 0.223. As Figure 4D, we show the 2nd degree MML fit for the low risk pooled MA, NJ and MO-IIa negative responding sets. The coefficients are a = 0.94, b = -4.69 E-02, c = 8.07 E-06, with an adjusted R^2 = 0.326. Again we see a best fit curve in Figure 37C that resembles the Representative alpha Particle Dose Response shape in Figure 10 of Part I. For both the Darby et al (2005, 2006) plus China (Blot et al 1990) and Krewski et al (2005, 2006) plus MA (Thompson et al 2008), we see the non-linear downward concave behavior expected for Bystander Damage predicted by the microdose BaD Model [Equation (2) and Figure 3 of Part I].

3.4 The Fit of the Case-Control Lung Cancer Studies Data for MA, NJ and MO-IIa to the Microdose Model

Using the original basic Microdose Model for Adaptive Response radio-protection (Leonard 2007a), it has been shown, with some examples given above in Figure 17 in Part II, for numerous Adaptive Response behaving dose response data sets (Leonard 2008b), that when AR is activated by a Poisson distributed single low LET induced charged particle tracks through each cell, the AR protection dominates the response with a dose response level below the zero dose level or below a Relative Risk of unity in the AR Microdose Model Equation (3) in Part II. It would be very significant if radon induced human lung cancer is indeed sensitive to Adaptive Response radio-protection mechanisms from the low LET natural background and man-made human

117

radiation exposures. For this reason, in our study it was important to examine any possible direct correlation providing evidence of this. To date, no justifiable reason has been shown for the very large variation in the incidence of human lung cancer with residential radon levels based on the case-control studies as we have shown in Figures 35A through 35F.

Figure 38 - Adaptive Response Micodose Model fit to MA (Panel A and Panel B), NJ (Panel C and Panel D) and MO-IIa (Panel E and Panel F) data

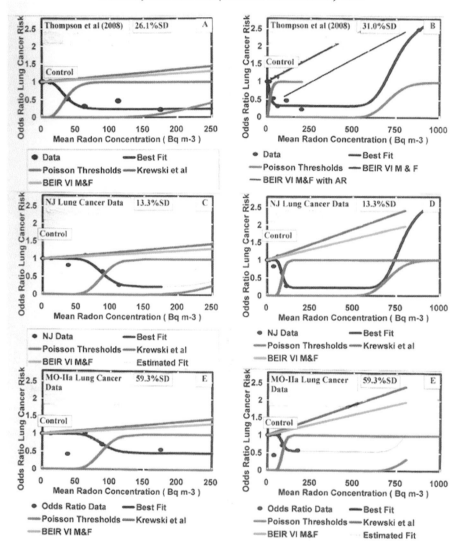

Figure 38 - Adaptive Response Micodose Model fit to MA (Panel A and Panel B), NJ (Panel C and Panel D) and MO-IIa (Panel E and Panel F) data (Krewski et al 2005, 2006). Shown are the Poisson Thresholds for activation of the adaptive response protection and the linear slopes from Krewski et al (2005, 2006) and the BEIR VI (1999) Lung Cancer Relative Risk.

We, in Figures 38A through 38F, show the use of the original basic Adaptive Response Microdose Model [Equation (3) of Part II] to evaluate Adaptive Response radio-protection as a possible and probable cause of the non-linear, "U" shaped negative response seen in the MA, NJ and MO-IIa data. Shown in the fits are the linearized dose response as predicted by the BEIR VI (1999) Report (slope 0.19 per 100 Bq m^{-3}) and the linearized response obtained by Krewski et al (2005) (slope 0.176 per 100 Bq m^{-3}). We have used a linear coefficient of 0.00176 for the α in Equation (3) of Part II i.e. α = 0.00176 lung cancers per Bq m^{-3} of radon. Shown are two graphs for each of the MA, NJ and MO-IIa data for low radon exposure levels to 250 Bq m^{-3} and for a high radon range showing the transition to a linear response dictated by the value of α. Referring to Figure 2 of Part II and the three damage regions, Bystander Effect Region, Adaptive Response Region and Direct Damage Region that were so useful in evaluation of AR protection for mammogram and diagnostic X-rays (Leonard and Leonard 2008), for lack of data, we simply estimated the Direct Damage threshold and transition to the high radon linear region. We also assumed that at high radon levels that the Adaptive Response protection is dissipated i.e. $f(M) \rightarrow 0$ in Equation (3) of Part II as observed in earlier evaluated data. There are not enough data to distinguish between AR protection for the spontaneous, priming dose and radon cancer incidence. As discussed in detail in Leonard (2008b), this has been the case for other Microdose Model analysis. Also, the data is insufficient to detect any possible very low level Bystander Effect, either deleterious or protective [although the low part of the negative responses could be protective Bystander as observed in Leonard (2008a, 2008b)]. The resolved best fit parameters, to $\pm 31\%$SD, for MA in Figures 38A and 38B are: S related to a threshold of 34 Bq m^{-3}, $P_{prot-pr\infty}$ = 0.76 (76% AR protection) and α = 0.00176 per Bq m^{-3} [note that the Thompson et al (2008) $\geq$ 250 Bq m^{-3} data point provides a good fit to α]. For NJ in Figure 38C and 38D, the resolved best fit parameters, $\pm 11\%$SD, are: S is related to a threshold of 80 Bq m^{-3}, $P_{prot-s\infty}$ = 0.49 (49% AR protection) and assumed α = 0.00176 per Bq m^{-3}. For MO-IIa in Figures 38E and 38F, the resolved parameters, to $\pm 10\%$SD, are: S related to a threshold of 82 Bq m^{-3}, $P_{prot-s\infty}$ = 0.78 (78% AR protection) and assumed α = 0.00176 per Bq m^{-3}. We use the term "related to" for the values of S since in Appendix A of Part II. We have shown a possible correlation between low LET external terrestrial, internal Radon progeny beta and ^{40}K and external cosmic radiations. What is apparent, from these case-control data analysis presented here, is that the data show that there must be more than just the Linear No-Threshold dose response mechanism affecting human lung cancer risks. This other mechanism must be the protective mechanism provided by the

119

Adaptive Response effect as a result of the wide variation in geological and ecological conditions existing worldwide as shown by the large variations in natural background and man-made radiations predicted in Section 3.1 and Figures 23 through 28.

4. ANALYSIS

4.1 Recent Case-Control Studies and Pooled Data – Variability of Human Lung Cancer Risks from Radon

We have used Figures 35A through 35F to show the very large range of results, fit to a linear model, for the European pooled data of Darby et al (2005, 2006) and Shengyang, China (Blot et al 1990) (Figure 35A – 35C) data and the North American pooled data of Krewski et al (2005, 2006) and Thompson et al (2008) (Figures 35D – 35F). Due to the very large variations in the linear fits to both pooled data sets, we have used the Papworth (1975) Poisson Validation Test to statistically analyze the data We refer to the Poisson Validation Test relative to Papworth because he was one of the first to propose the Method of Maximum Likelihood procedure for fitting experimental data and the Poisson Test to validate the data sets (Papworth 1975, Savage and Papworth 2000, Edwards et al 1979). The Papworth Poisson Validation Test indicated that both the pooled data of Krewski et al (2005, 2006) and Darby et al (2005, 2006) to be over-dispersed and assessed to be "contaminated" by other auxiliary influences, as shown in Figure 36. Allowing for non-linearity, without a presumption that it be from Adaptive Response radio-protection, we have then used MML to trial fit to all the data sets to 3rd, 4th and 5th degree polynomials, $a + bX + cX^2 + dX^3 + eX^4 + fX^5$, showing considerable non-linearity. These polynomial fits are shown in Figure 37 showing very significant resemblance to the non-linear Representative Alpha Particle Dose Response shape of Figure 10 of Part I and in particular the Bystander Damage Region. As we noted above, in the pooling of data from these studies, the pool participants basically applied a crucial assumption that between-site differences seen in the observed relationship between lung cancer risk and radon exposure are due to random measurement variability and the true relationship is independent of site locality and only dependent on the carcinogenic sensitivity of human lung tissue to alpha radiation (which is assumed to be an invariant and Linear with No-Threshold). The polynomial fits to these case-control data conclusively shows that their assumption is invalid. The fit of the original basic AR Microdose Model, in Figure 38, to the negative responding data from the MA, NJ and MO-IIa studies indicates that there is negligible lung cancer risks and the presence of a

120

dominating Adaptive Response radio-protection from any radon progeny inducing lung cancer and naturally occurring spontaneous (non-radon) lung cancers.

As Figure 39, we examine the polynomial fits to the high risk groups for the Darby et al (2005, 2006) and the Krewski et al (2005, 2006) data. The Figure 39A Darby et al (2005, 2006) high risk group polynomial fit shows very similar characteristics to the alpha particle dose response data analyzed in Chapter 2 - Part I, the Representative Alpha Particle Dose Response shape curves in Figure 10 and the composite BE and AR Microdose Model estimates in Figures 33 and 34 considering Adaptive Response protection from lung cancer from natural background and man-made radiations. We thus label the three response regions i.e. Bystander Damage Region, Threshold Region and Direct Damage Region as we have done in our other BE and AR studies (Leonard 2008a, 2008b, Leonard and Leonard 2008). Two areas are worthy of noting as 1 and 2 on the Figure 39A graph. Area 1 shows the a flat region in the beginning caused by the lowest radon category, where most values are 1.00, designated as slightly above zero radon, but technically should be considered as a data point at zero radon level. Correlating with the representative Figure 8, Part I curve, the area 2 is most likely the single to double alpha traversal threshold and transition region into the Direct Damage Region (see Section 4.1.a of Part I). We have included in the graph the curve from Figure 32A, Part II (as "BE Microdose Model"), which is the estimated Relative Lung Cancer Risk at the UNSCEAR (2000) worldwide average human background, low LET exposure. Significantly, the Figure 32A, Part II curve was shifted slightly to provide a good correlation and gives an indication of the radon concentration level that the radon cancer Direct Damage begins in the dose response. Figure 39B provides the high risk group polynomial fit from the pooled North American (Krewski et al 2005, 2006) data. Their data points only extend to 250 Bq m^{-3}, so they provide just the Bystander Damage Region cancer risk. Figure 39C shows, with both the Darby et al (2005, 2006) plus China (Blot et al 1990) and Krewski et al (2005, 2006) plus MA (Thompson et al 2008) high risks fits, that the two are in extremely good agreement.

Figure 38, The polynomial Method of Maximum Likelihood fits to the high risk group's data for both the Krewski et al plus MA and the Darby et al plus China data

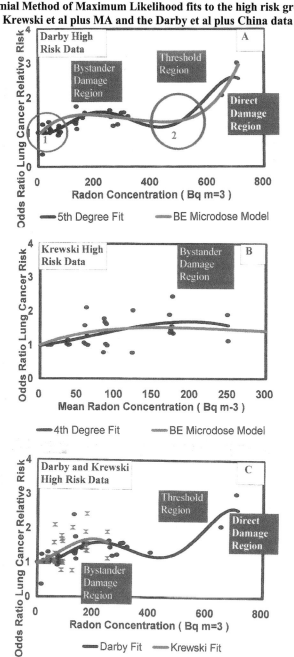

Figure 39 - The polynomial Method of Maximum Likelihood fits to the high risk groups data for both the Krewski et al plus MA and the Darby et al plus China data. Panel A – The 5th degree polynomial fit to both the Darby/China high risk group data. The circled area, labeled "1" is the low region where the low data shows minimal increase in risk. The area labeled "2" is most probably where the Threshold and Transition to the Direct Damage response occurs. The Darby high and low risk groups required 5th degree polynomial fits. Panel B - The Krewski et al plus MA high risk group data fit to a 3rd degree polynomial. Only a 3rd degree fit was needed since the data extends only to within the Bystander Damage Region to 250 Bq m-3 Panel C – The 5th degree fit of all Darby/China and Krewski/MA data.

The two low risk data groups polynomial fits are shown in Figures 37C and 37E. The low risk fit for the North American (Krewski et al 2005, 2006) data for MA, NJ and MO-IIa, in Figure 38, show a very large Adaptive Response protection and no resemblance of a Bystander Damage Region, Threshold Region or Direct Damage Region (although the Direct Damage would not be seen for the highest 250 Bq m⁻³ data points). This suggests a complete Adaptive Response protection that negates the alpha particle lung damage, but further provides beneficial protection from naturally occurring, spontaneous (non-radon) lung cancer risk from endogenic toxic chromosome damage or hereditary lung cancers (since they are lower than the zero radon concentration risks). The Darby et al (2005, 2006) low risk data fit shown in Figure 37C, which includes Western Germany, Spain, Finland nationwide and China, shows the same characteristics of a combined Bystander and AR protection as the Figure 37B for the high risk data but lower in lung cancer risk but also concave downward.

Figure 39, Analysis of the MML polynomial fits

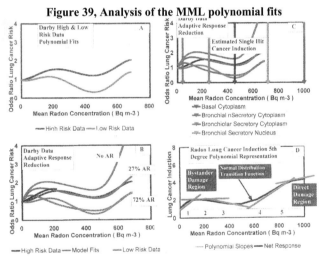

Figure 40 - Analysis of the MML polynomial fits. Panel A – Shown are the high and low risk group fits for the Darby/China data. Both curves show the behavior depicted by the Representative Shape Microdose Model in Figure 10 of Part I. The lower curve is from reduction of cancer risk by Adaptive Response suppression. Panel B – We show the Representative Shape from Figure 10 of Part I superposition on the high risk data fits. Here we show that the Darby/China low risk curve also conforms to the same shape behavior but at further reduced levels. We estimates the relative lung cancer risk. The top curve would be with no Adaptive Response protection, The two middle curves are the observed high risk and low risk Darby/China fits showing relative Adaptive Response protection. Panel C – The polynomial fits to the case-control data show excellent agreement with the Representative Shape composite Bystander and Adaptive Response Microdose Model given in Figure 10 of Part I, which is primarily based on relative chromosome aberration incidence rates. The "U" shaped behavior of the case-control data provides an indication of the radon concentration at which the single hit occurs for lung cancer induction. James et al provides estimates of the correlation between single alpha particle traversals per kBq m-3 of indoor radon exposure per 30 lung cell mitotic cycle. They provide data for both the nucleus and separately the entire cell (cytoplasm hits). It would be expected that this single hit cancer induction level,

shown to be at about 490 Bq m-3, would be greater than the James et al values. We show in Panel C the James et al radon concentration single hit values for the indicated traversals for the indicated lung cells. Only the single hits for the Bronchial and Bronchiolar Secretory cells are below the Estimated Single Hit Cancer Induction concentration. This suggests that the sensitive volume for the human lung cells for lung cancer induction may be the entire cell. Based on the Adaptive Response analysis presented in Appendix B and Section 3.2, all data groups suggest some AR protection i.e. the Darby and Krewski high risk groups 27%, the Darby low group about 72% protection and the Krewski low group about 100% protections. Panel D – Illustration as to why a 3rd degree polynomial was adequate for the Krewski/MA fit and a 5th degree polynomial was needed for the Darby/China data. In the Bystander Damage Region the concave curvature is easily fit with 3 different slopes, whereas for the Darby/China data extending to the Direct Damage Region the three Bystander Region slopes are needed but a slope for the Threshold, the Transition and the final Direct Damage slope.

To compare the two further, we show them together in Figure 40A where we see a distinctly greater Adaptive Response protection for the low risk group (as would be expected). In Figure 40B, we show fits to the Figure 10 Representative Alpha Particle Dose Response shape curve but imposing an additional AR protection reduction seen by the blue solid curves. Although somewhat confusing, we show the high risk curve for the equivalent Darby et al (2005, 2006) and Krewski et al (2005, 2006) data (solid black) and the Darby et al (2005, 2006) low risk curve (solid red) together in Figure 40C, indicating various degrees of Adaptive Response protection as compared to the risk without any AR protection (top curve). Based on our calculations in Chapter 3 - Part II, we estimate that the high Darby et al (2005, 2006) and Krewski et al (2005, 2006) data show some Adaptive Response radio-protection of about 27%. For the low Darby et al (2005, 2006) data there is an AR protection of about 72% and for the low Krewski et al (2005, 2006) plus MA (Thompson et al 2008) data the protection is about 100%. In Panel D of Figure 40, we show for the Darby et al (2005, 2006) data why a 5th degree polynomial was required for the best fit. Five different slopes were encompassed in the fit to the Odds Ratio data.

4.2 Summary of Part III

We have analyzed the data from the North American (Krewski et al 2005, 2006) pooled study, the European (Darby et al 2005, 2006) pooled study, the Massachusetts (Thompson et al 2008) study and the China (Blot et al 1990). The North American study included 3662 lung cancer cases and 4966 controls. The European study included 7148 cases and 14269 controls. Altogether our analysis encompassed over 11000 cases and 20000 controls. By applying the Papworth (1975) Poisson Validation Test for linear correlation it is shown that the basic premises of Krewski et al (2005, 2006) and Darby et al (2005, 2006) that "between-site differences seen in the observed relationship between lung cancer risk and radon exposure are due to random measurement variability and the true relationship is independent of site locality and only dependent on the carcinogenic sensitivity of human lung tissue to alpha radiation" in conclusively invalid. Case-control studies show zero and negative lung cancer risks with increasing human radon exposure. By dividing the studies into two groups, those showing positive risks (high groups) and those showing zero or negative risks (low groups), polynomial fits were performed to the data. The curves obtained for the high and low Darby et al (2005, 2006) groups (Figures 37A and 37B) displayed non-coincidental, strong similarity to the expected curves obtained from Figures 10 and 16 of Part I and Figures 32, 33 and 34 reflecting Bystander and Adaptive Response behavior. The Chapter 3 - Part II expected curves were derived from the Bystander BaD Model, reflecting primarily Bystander Damage as the inductive damage for domestic and workplace radon lung cancers. The polynomial fit for the Krewski et al (2005, 2006) high group matched that for the Darby et al (2005, 2006) high group and the fit to the low Krewski et al (2005, 2006) group showed no radon lung cancer risk and a large reduction in the zero radon natural spontaneous risks. In Figure 40B, we estimate an Adaptive Response reduction of about 27% for the Darby et al (2005, 2006) and Krewski et al (2005, 2006) high groups, about a 72% AR reduction for the low Darby et al (2005, 2006) group and a 100% AR reduction for the Krewski et al (2005, 2006) low group.

Chapter 5 - ANALYSIS AND CONCLUSIONS FROM PARTS I, II AND III

New Evidence About the Cellular Sensitive Volume for Human Lung Cancer Induction From Radon

We have cited the recent reassessment of the alpha particle dosimetry for the BEIR VI (1999) report by James et al (2004) in Part I. The important 30 day lung cell mitotic cycle single particle hit probabilities are given in their Table 12. The ICRP (1994) Report 66 values as given in James et al (2004) Table 12 are 0.36, 1.4 and 0.51 hits per Basal, Bronchial Secretrory and Bronchiolar Secretory cells respectively per kBq m^{-3} of radon for cell nucleus hits and 1.0, 16, and 4.0 hits per Basal, Bronchial Secretrory and Bronchiolar Secretory cells respectively per kBq m^{-3} of radon for cell cytoplasm hits (entire cell as "target"). As Figure 4 of Part I, we have provided graphs of the variation in single alpha hit probabilities for the three primarily alpha induced cancer sensitive cells in the lung i.e. the Bronchial Basal, the Bronchial Secretory and the Bronchiolar Secretory cells. In Figure 13 of Chapter 2 - Part I, we provide the correlation between radon concentrations and Specific Energy Hits for these three cell species for the nucleus and entire cell volumes relative to the Representative alpha Particle Dose Response shape response. In Figure 15 of Chapter 2 - Part I, we show the alpha traversal rates for the BEIR VI (1999) radon concentration frequency distribution in US homes and in Figure 12 of Part I, we show the sensitive cells hit rates for the BEIR VI (1999), Figure 3-2 lung cancer relative risks. The Figure 40, Panels A, B and C show that the "U" shaped Direct Damage Threshold and Transition Region occurs at a radon concentration of about 450 Bq m^{-3}. This radon concentration value then can be deemed as approximately the single to double hit transition for Direct Damage lung cancer induction concentration. In Figure 40C, we show this accordingly as the "Estimated Single Hit Cancer Induction" level. From the analysis of the alpha particle micro-beam and broad-beam data in Appendix A of Part I, we developed a Representative Alpha Particle Dose Response shape in Figure 10 of Chapter 2 - Part I which we felt typifies alpha particle produced neoplastic transformation and chromosome aberration production for the 6.00 and 7.69 MeV radon progeny alphas. We have marked the Bronchial Secretory cytroplasm, the Bronchiolar Secretory cytoplasm, the Bronchial Secretory nucleus and the Basal cytoplasm on the Figure 40C graph, from James et al (2004) Table 12. In Figure 10 of Chapter 2 - Part I, we have also provided different abscissa scales for conversion to effective radon concentrations for hits to the three sensitive cells and separately as to whether the nucleus or the cytoplasm are hit in the 30 day mitotic cycle. The Basal nucleus and Bronchiolar Secretory nucleus are 2778 Bq m^{-3} and 1960 Bq m^{-3} and would be off scale on the Figure 40C graph. By basic definition of the Direct Damage Region and the Direct Damage Threshold, we would expect that one or more alpha particle traversals to occur to produce the threshold for Direct Damage production of lung cancer in humans. We would expect that the radon concentration for the single hits per kBq m^{-3} values to fall below the estimated lung cancer single hit lung cancer induction value in the "U" shaped region. We therefore must significantly conclude that either the estimated single hit values for nucleus traversals from ICRP (1994) Report 66 and James et al (2004) are incorrect or the sensitive "target" for lung cancer induction is larger than just the cell nucleus. Wu et al (1999) and Shao et al (2008) have observed induction of Bystander responses by targeting the cytoplasm. Based on Figure 40C, our analysis of the case-control studies supports their work that the sensitive cell volume for lung cancer induction in humans may be the entire cell of the three sensitive lung cell species.

Mechanisms and Responses for a Non-Linear Human Lung Cancer Risk

We have shown that most probably there is a significant role of the Adaptive Response radio-protective mechanism in explaining the very large variation in dose response results for human lung cancer risk from case-control studies world-wide. Leonard (2008b) extensively reviews the data showing that low LET radiation induced, Poisson distributed, single charged particle traversals through target cells activates the protective mechanism against potentially carcinogenic, exogenic large radiation challenge dose damage and also against non-radon, endogenic, toxic, naturally occurring, spontaneous chromosome damage. Past and current radiobiology research results can not offer any other plausible explanation for this large variation without completely discounting the case-control concept as a valid cancer research tool, which is strongly supported by BEIR VI (1999). The radon progeny alpha particle damage can be viewed as exogenic challenge dose damage when Adaptive Response protection is present. The fact that some case-control data, such as the MA, NJ and MO-IIa data, show a reduction below the zero radon, natural spontaneous level means that the human low LET background and man-made radiations also provide protection against the endogenic toxic spontaneous chromosome damage in the lung tissue.

127

Much is not known to explain the protective behavior. It is well confirmed that single traversals activate AR. Redpath and Elmore (2007) report that the Reactive Oxygen Species concentration is reduced during AR protection, so perhaps the very small amount of free radicals from the single traversal, produces a bio-chemical warning and activates the production of cell chemicals that quench the spontaneous and radiation produced radicals such as hydrogen peroxide. It is known that in AR protection ATM is activated and a G2 arrest is initiated. The distinction between the type of chromosome damages by the Bystander signals and from direct alpha hits are not clearly known. Also, is there a distinction between the type chromosome damage from an alpha particle traversal through the cell nucleus and the cytoplasm? Cancer development involves a multi-stage process so the off-set between the alpha particle hit rates and cancer induction suggested in Figure 40C may be reconciled.

Chapter 6 - DISCUSSION

Use of the Papworth (1975) Poisson Validation Test

One can argue that it is inappropriate to apply the Papworth (1975) Poisson Validation Test to the case-control data by use of the risk data points variation from the linearized slope curve, which is a continuous function of radon concentration. In Section 3.2, we have argued here that the very large case and control populations in our study justifies the invalidation of the assumption of BEIR VI and the Darby and Krewski that the linearized curve represents a very accurate quantitative estimate of the "true relationship (between human lung cancer risk and radon concentration) independent of site locality".

Validity of *In vitro* Dose Response Studies in Predicting *In vivo* Radiation Effects

Most of the dose response data examined here with respect to the Bystander and Adaptive Response Effects are *in vitro* from cell culture studies of others. There is always the question of validity of *in vitro* cellular dose response results, when applied to anticipated radiation dose response in humans. Tissue cultures first came into use in the study of radiation dose response relative to cancer radiation therapy. For radio-therapy, of particular concern was the cell killing radiosensitivity and cell recovery (repair) capability of tumor and peripheral tissue and organs. In the 1970s with newly developed *in vitro* cellular techniques, the research group at Columbia University directed by Dr. Eric Hall (Hall 2000) performed *in vitro* dose and dose rate dependent studies of a number of new mammalian cell species. Dr. Halls (Hall 2000) group was meticulous to obtain many different dose rates data sets with dose rate data as low as 10 cGy h^{-1}. These data were found to be useful in our "Inverse" Dose Rate Effect studies (Leonard 2000, 2007a, Leonard and Lucas 2008, 2009). The cell species studied were V79 log phase, V79 plateau phase, HeLa log phase, C3H 10T1/2 plateau phase, C3H 10T1/2 log phase, CHF-F log phase, rat kangaroo, Munt Jac, pig kidney and L-P59 cells. As more human *in vitro* cell strains became available, *in vitro* dose rate response studies were possible with direct human application to continuous protracted (brachytherapy) and fractionated radiotherapy. Thus, in the 1980s, there were dose and dose rate surviving fraction *in vitro* dose response measurements on numerous human cell tissues, many of them by Dr.

Gordon Steel (Steel et al 1987) and his radio-biology research group. In a review article by Steel et al (1987), the dose response of human tumor cell lines were summarized i.e. HX34 melanoma, RT112 bladder, HX118 melanoma, HX142 neuroblastoma, HX156 cervix carcinoma, HX138 neuroblastoma, GCT27 testis, HX58 pancreas, WX67 bladder and HX143 neuroblastoma.

In support of the Hall (Hall 2000) and Steel (Steel et al 1987) groups work, the dose and dose rate dependent analytical models of Thames (1985) (Incomplete Repair - IR) and Curtis (1986) (Lethal Potential Lethal – LPL) Models (see Table II Steel et al 1987) were developed. Only two or three separate dose rates were sufficient to determine the α (single hit L-Q damage rate per unit dose), the β (double hit L-Q damage rate per square of dose) and the mean repair half-time, $T_{1/2}$ (in hours). A more complete list of these parameters for 38 cells of human origin is provided in Table 1 of Brenner and Hall (1991). Small numbers of dose rate data sets were adequate to determine these three parameters. For example in terms of dose rate data sets, Kelland and Steel (1986) provided data for four human tumors with only two dose rates (acute 150 cGy/min and 1.6 cGy/min) for HX58 and HX32 (both pancreatic carcinoma) and only three dose rates (acute 1.50 Gy/min, 7.6 cGy/min and 1.6 cGy/min) for HX118 melanoma and HX99 breast carcinoma. Similarly, McMillan et al (1989) provided two dose rate data sets for the human neuroblastoma cells HX142 and HX138 (acute 1.8 Gy/min and 1 cGy/min). Cassoni et al (1992) obtained only two dose rate data sets for four human lung carcinomas (two small-cell and two non-small cell, HC12, HX149, HX147A7 and HX148G7. Stephens et al (1987) provided 4 dose rate data sets for HX34 human melanoma and 6 data sets for MT mouse mammary carcinoma which we were able to use with their isodose curves in our earlier studies (Leonard 2000, 2007a) as non-IDRE responding cells. Furre et al (1999) only provided three dose rate data sets for the human cervix carcinoma cell line NHIK 3025, but fortunately the lowest dose rate data set at 33 cGy h^{-1} showed a significant hyper-radiosensitivity as compared to a higher dose rate of 94 cGy h^{-1}.

There are several tools, developed in the late 1980's and 1990's, that have been used by radiotherapists for evaluation of human tissue dose rate effects primarily for low dose rate (LDR) and high dose rate (HDR) brachytherapy treatments and high dose rate fractionation. They are first the isoeffect dose rate curves for constant surviving fraction which were utilized early in radiotherapy analysis. The second major tool was the dose and dose rate dependent cell radiation response models cited above. From these modeling sources, various parameters are obtained from fit of these models to laboratory measured *in vitro* dose rate response data i.e. α / β ratios for the linear-quadratic model and the biological effective dose (BED) (Jones et al 2001). Due to dose rate effects, it has been known that there is a therapeutic advantage between tumor control and normal tissue complications for fractionation or protraction (brachytherapy). For example, it has been found that typically high α / β ratios, determined from model fitting to *in vitro* data, are characteristic of normal peripheral tissues that show an early deleterious response in fractionated treatments (see Chapter 22, Hall 2000). Recent analysis of α / β ratios for prostate carcinoma cells are reported (Brenner et al 2002, Carlson et al 2004) that show low α / β ratios and high radio-sensitivity similar to late responding tissue. In Figure 3 of Brenner (1997), a distinction is made between early responding and late responding human tissues (steeper slopes) using isoeffect curves for brachytherapy as well as for fractionation. *In vitro* cellular dose response measurements and the application of the BED, IR and LPL Models are still extensively used in radio-therapy treatment planning (Hall 2000, Brenner et al 2002, Jones et al 2001).

Hyper-radiosensitivity to cell-killing at very low doses was first observed from *in vitro* cellular dose response data and is now extensively studied with respect to radio-therapy of solid tumor treatment (Marples et al 2004). This effect has been labeled Hyper-Radiosensitivity and Induced Radio-Resistance (HRS/IRR). It has been found, with the *in vitro* studies, that about 80% of cell species studied (Dasu and Denekamp 2000) experience HRS/IRR. This is found to be true for 45 human cell species (Joiner et al 2001). In radiotherapy, this very low dose hyper-radiosensitivity is being examined for possible therapeutic gain by the use of ultra-fractionated dose from 0.5 to 1.5 Gy instead of the fractionated doses of 2.0 Gy in conventional radiotherapy treatment regimes (Slonina et al 2007, Harney et al 2004a, 2004b). Conclusive *in vitro* benefits for head and neck cancers have been shown and potential benefits for brain glioma cancers are suggested (Dey et al 2003, Tome and Howard 2007). The University of Kentucky Markey Cancer Center has recruited head and neck tumor patients for a bi-weekly combined gemcitabine and paclitaxel and low-dose radiation treatment program using 50 to 80 cGy twice daily (4 hours apart) radiation exposures (see internet *ClinicalTrials.gov Identifier NCT00176241*). From *in vitro* data correlating IDRE with the HRS/IRR hyper-radiosensitivity (Leonard 2000, 2007d), it is suggested that the "Inverse" Dose Rate

Effect hyper-radiosensitivity may cause excessive cell killing in LDR brachytherapy of preferential tissues and organs but also may have a therapeutic gain if tumor cells undergo IDRE (Leonard and Lucas 2008, 2009).

In the last 25 years, on the order of thousands of oncogenic neoplastic transformation and chromosome aberration *in vitro* studies have been reported with the presumption of a correlation of *in vitro* data with human carcinogenesis. Based on the extensive studies of *in vitro* alpha particle cellular dose response to ionizing radiations (Miller et al 1995, 1999, Zhou et al 2001, 2004, Nagasawa and Little 1999, 2002, Nagasawa et al 2003, Hei et al 1997, Sawant et al 2001) and analyzed in Part I, there has been a presumption that the Bystander Effect is experienced by humans in the induction of radon induced lung cancer (Zhou et al 2001, Brenner et al 2001, Brenner and Sachs 2002, Little and Wakeford 2001, Little 2004). The extensive Adaptive Response *in vitro* research cited here (Azzam et al 1996, Elmore et al 2006, 2008, Ko et al 2004, Redpath et al 2001, 2003, Redpath and Antoniono 1998, Shadley and Wiencke 1989, Shadley and Wolff 1987, Shadley et al 1987, Wiencke et al 1986, Wolff et al 1989, 1991) and analyzed with the composite AR and BE Microdose Model (Leonard 2005, 2007a, 2007b, 2008a, 2008b, Leonard and Leonard 2008) is supportive of humans experiencing Adaptive Response radio-protection from low LET radiation exposures. As shown in the next section, there are more *in vivo* relatively new data supporting AR protection than BE damage in humans. It is generally accepted that the induction of carcinogenesis in the human anatomy can be predictable by *in vitro* observation of cellular damage mechanisms.

In vivo Examples of Adaptive Response Radio-protective Dose Response to Ionizing Radiations

Although we have in the previous section given examples of how *in vitro* dose response data have assisted radio-biologist and radio-therapist in anticipating human dose response to radiation and suggested that these data support a premise of *in vitro* data that there are Bystander and Adaptive Response effects in humans, some critics have noted that little *in vivo* data are available. We offer the following relatively recent *in vivo* results. A number of animal laboratory exposures to ionizing radiations have shown the ability of cells, tissues and organs to exhibit Adaptive Response radio-protection from low doses. There are also some examples of AR reduction effects for human exposures. We here cite a few of these cases. Perhaps the most directly applicable case to AR reduction in lung cancer incidence is the analysis conducted by Rossi and Zaider (1997) of about 14,000 women that had received radio-therapy treatment for breast cancer (we show their dose response data as Figure 41A, reproduced from Figure 3B of Leonard (2007a).

Figure 40, Examples of reduction in lung cancer incidence below the zero-radon spontaneous level

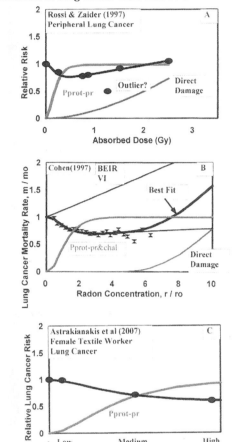

Figure 41 - Examples of reduction in lung cancer incidence below the zero-radon spontaneous level. The red curves show the estimated Poisson distributed Adaptive Response activation. Panel A – The data of Rossi and Zaider (1997) (Rossi 1999) of reduction in lung cancer for women treated for breast cancer with radio-therapy. Panel B = The epidemiological data of Cohen (1997) of lung cancer incidence by counties in the US. Panel C - The observed lung cancer risk in a case=control study of textile workers in Shanghai, China exposed to toxic textile chemicals.

The epidemiological data of Cohen (1997), presented here as Figure 41B, showing a reduction in lung cancer incidence in the US with increasing radon levels, has generated 20 years of controversy. His response curve is even shown in the BEIR VI (1999) Figure 3-2 reproduced in our Figures 1C and 15 OF Part I. Two non-radiation case-control studies (Levin et al 1987, Astrakianakis et al 2007), the data shown in Figure 41C for textile workers in Shanghai, China, found a reduction in lung cancer risk of about

133

30% with increasing endotoxin exposure. The first study involved 1405 cancer cases and 1495 controls. Dr. Blot, who did the Shengyang, China radon case-control study (Blot et al 1990), was a participant in this study. The more recent study involved 628 cancer cases and 3184 controls. These AR reduction findings are similar to that of US textile workers (Henderson and Enterline 1973). Although the studies did not involve radiation as the toxigen, it does suggest an ability of lung tissue to activate protective mechanisms under stress conditions.

The most recent, and believed to be most significant, studies have been with live whole-body exposures of mice. Wang and Cai (2000) irradiated live mice to a 6 Gy challenge dose and found that with administering a priming dose of 0.5 Gy 48 hours prior to the challenge dose, the effect on red blood count, white blood count and platelet count was reduced by 90%. Day et al (2006) exposed live pKZ1 mice prostate gland to challenge doses of 1000 mGy of X-rays and measured the chromosome inversion frequency. By pre-exposing the mice to very low doses of X-rays (0.001 to 10 mGy), a reduction of from 50 to 70% was observed with the greatest reduction for the 0.001 mGy exposure. Two research groups have examined the effect of low dose rate exposures, at rates comparable to human dose rates. Ina and Sakai (2005) exposed MRL-lpr/lpr mice to a chronic dose rate of 1.2 mGy/h for a series of prolonged exposure experiments and studied the life-span effect. For life-long exposures, they observed what has to be considered a remarkable result. The median life-span of 134 days of unexposed mice was extended to 502 days from these continuous exposures. At the dose rate used the exposed mice received the equivalent annual NRC permitted dose for nuclear workers in 2 days, and yet they survived for 502 days. With a series of experiments with cancer proned, Trp53 heterozygous mice, the dose rates were at levels that occupational nuclear workers would be expected to receive under normal work conditions at sub-NRC levels.

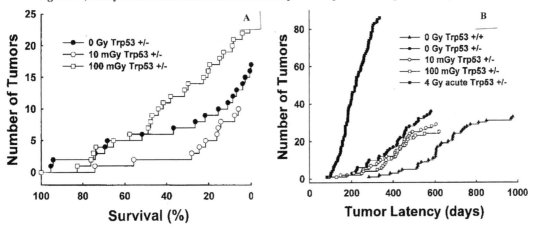

Figure 42 – In vivo studies of low dose rate induction of Adaptive Response radio-protection (Mitchel et al 2003). Panel A – The appearance of spinal osteosarcomas associated with paralysis in Trp53 heterozygous mice (+/-) at low occupational level dose rate. Panel B – Tumor latency of lymphomas appearing in unexposed Trp53 normal (+/+) and Trp53 heterozygous (+/-) mice exposed to indicated doses of 60Co radiation.

What has been shown is that for these mice *in vivo*, such low doses induce an Adaptive Response that increases tumor latency and increases the life span as shown in Figures 42A and 42B (from Mitchel et al 2003). These data show the Adaptive Response radio-protection from endogenic, spontaneous, genetically inheritable tumor development. A low-dose threshold exists for the Adaptive Response protection against chronic ulcerative dermatitis, a spontaneous, autoimmune-type age-related disease in the C57BL/6 mice (Mitchel 2007b). For that non-cancer disease, these very low-dose fractionated exposures induced a protective Adaptive Response in both Trp53 normal and heteroztgous mice, but a lower threshold level of exposure had to be exceeded. This shows that low doses of low LET radiation can activate tumor protective mechanisms, but with a minimum threshold, just as we have seen in the *in vitro* AR data in Figure 1 of Part II and our other work. But also, there is a high dose threshold where the Direct Damage dominates the AR protection., as also we have seen in our analysis of the *in vitro* data and shown in Figure 21A of Chapter 3 - Part II at around 10 cGy of priming dose. Dr. Mitchel refers to this as an Adaptive Response "Dose Window" and discusses this in a recent paper (Mitchel 2010).

Some Special Considerations Relative to the Combined Bystander and Adaptive Response Lung Dose Response

In a recent Dose-Response Journal review article (Leonard 2008b), the various circumstances under which Adaptive Response protection can be experienced was presented. In Section 2.3 of Chapter 3 - Part II, we have summarized key AR responding data relative to protection from large "challenge" doses of radiation and from naturally occurring, potentially carcinogenic, spontaneous cellular damage. What occurs in the human lung from radon progeny alpha particles can be perceived as alpha particle "challenge" dose damage, which we have shown is modulated by the AR from the continual human low LET exposures. In the laboratory, a "challenge" dose experiment, such as those performed by the Shadley, Wiencke and Wolff research group (Shadley and Wiencke 1989, Shadley and Wolff 1987, Shadley et al 1987, Wiencke et al 1986, Wolff et al 1989, 1991), is with a single large "challenge" dose exposure. In assessing human cancer risk from radon, we are examining a continuum of exposure data over a wide range of alpha particle exposures to the lung. The analysis of the Pohl-Ruling (1988) radon exposure data involved a case where the radon progeny beta rays provided the low LET Adaptive Response protection [see Figure 4, Leonard (2008a)]. There then was a case of a continuum of beta ray AR protection with increasing radon exposure. We have included this beta source in our analysis here in Part II. We have also had to consider, in Part II, the variable increase in the Uranium terrestrial background radiation as a second continuum source to AR protection, thus resulting in increased AR protection with increasing domestic level human radon exposure.

Measurement of Indoor Gamma Ray Dose in Case-control Studies

The fact that underground miners lung cancer data may not be directly applicable to human lung cancer incidence at domestic and workplace radon levels, due to a distinct difference in cellular damage type from Bystander damage and direct cellular damage, means that case-control studies may be more significant in the assessment of lung cancer risks from radon. The evidence of Adaptive Response reduction of lung cancer risks from human exposure to low LET radio-protection suggests that planners for future case-control studies should consider the measurement of the indoor gamma and beta ray exposure levels as well as the radon concentration exposures in residences to assess AR protection. This would require portable gamma ray spectrometer systems. There are basically two type spectrometers that have been used. Clouvas et al (2001) used a high resolution Germanium solid state detector system that yields gamma spectrum data similar to that shown in Figure A1 of the Appendix A to Part II. The USGS and DOE aerial monitoring systems use a large NaI crystal as their detector (DOE 2002). This has a much higher detection efficiency than the much smaller Germanium detector and has been found to provide adequate resolution. The Germanium system requires then longer counting times to obtain a good spectrum. Portable automatic analyzer systems to resolve the individual gamma rays and their intensities are available for both.

Uncertainties in the Estimation of Combined BE and AR Effects on the Lung Cancer Risks from Radon

It has been found that the magnitude of the Adaptive Response protection below the zero priming dose response "challenge" damage or spontaneous damage level varies between about 50% to about 80%. This is shown by the research work of Redpaths group and analysis with our Microdose Model. We have here used a 65% reduction for the priming dose reduction parameter $P_{prot-pr}$ [see Equation (3) and then Appendix B for the definition]. The relative sensitivities of the three lung cell species to carcinogenesis is not accurately known (NRC 1991). It is suspected that the basal cells may have greater sensitivity than the other two, but not conclusively confirmed. We have here considered the three cells sensitivities as equal. There are uncertainties relative to the size of these cells as targets for charged particle traversal of both alphas and low LET traversals. We have used the BEIR VI (1999) values as have others (Little and Wakeford 2001, Brenner et al 2001, Little 2004, Brenner and Sachs 2002).

The compilation of lung cell Specific Energy traversals is conservative in that the external beta rays from the terrestrial radiations are not included, the 0.511 MeV annihilation gamma rays are neglected in the internal Potassium-40 activities, only the cosmic ray high energy protons are considered neglecting the approximately 10% high energy helium ions and neutrons and also any variation in Thorium terrestrial gammas with increasing radon concentration is neglected (USGS has only, so far, provided in the NURE report the Uranium terrestrial data). We have not considered any protective Bystander Effect even though there is evidence from recent work presented in Section 2.3.b and Figure 2 of Part II [and Leonard and Leonard (2008)]. Its presence would reduce the dose response at the very low dose region of the radon dose response curve.

In Figures 17 and 21A of Part II, it is shown that the domination of the Direct Damage component from priming doses in the Adaptive Response experiments begins at about 10 cGy of low LET primer dose. It is also shown throughout this work that the threshold for the Adaptive Response protection begins with a Poisson distributed mean single Specific Energy Hit. For the radiations tabulated in Table A1 of the Appendix A of Part II, this would occur on an average at about 0.10 cGy such that the Adaptive Response Region extends from about 0.10 cGy to about 10.0 cGy. With the UNSCEAR (2000) worldwide average human low LET exposure at about 1.7 mSv (see Table 1), a significant fraction of the human lung cells will have received to single low LET radiation induced charged particle traversal, activating the AR against the radon progeny alpha deleterious Bystander Damage. We show this from the Chapter 3 – Part II analysis.

The use of the modified BaD Model concave Bystander Damage dose response for the domestic region radon alpha induced Radon Lung Cancer Risk, without the presence of AR protection, provides an average for the domestic region, in Figure 13B of Part I, which is higher than provided by the approximately 0.0020 ERR/Bq m^{-3} BEIR VI (1999) estimate. For the radon range from zero to 400 Bq m^{-3} the average ERR using the concave Bystander Damage dose response in Figure 13B, Part I is 0.818 compared to the BEIR VI (1999) average ERR of 0.676 for the same range, meaning about a 20% higher lung cancer induction without AR protection being considered in the microbeam studies, which implies that the human body tissues always receives some Adaptive Response radio-protection since we always receive some background and man-made radiations.

We have shown that the 13 European case- control studies [plus the Blot et al (1990) study in Shenyang, China] and the 8 North American studies [plus the Thompson et al (2008) MA study] show such an extreme variation, that either the case-control methodology is totally invalid (which most radiobiologist and the BEIR committees are reluctant to premise) or that there are one or more other dose response mechanisms other than the Linear No-Threshold mechanism. It is significant to note that Krewski et al (2005, 2006), in their analysis of their study, indicates that if the Iowa data is removed from the North American pooling, then any statistically positive association between radon and lung cancer disappears [e.g. the dose response slope, beta (95% CL) in our Equation (C1), reduces to 0.04 (-0.04, 0.19) per 100 Bq m^{-3}] (see their page 578). Also, Darby et al (2005) shows no statistically significant Relative Risk below 100 Bq m^{-3} as compared to the reference value below 25 Bq m^{-3} (see their Table 2) and they suggest a possible threshold at 150 Bq m^{-3} (see their paragraph 1, page 224). There seems to be considerable uncertainty in their analysis and results. Another example is the case-control study in Spain where Darby et al (2005) reports a negative slope whereas the original publication (Barros et al 2002) reports a positive slope for beta in Equation (1) in Chapter 4 - Part III. The Spanish study of Llorca et al (2007) showing no correlation between radon and lung cancer was not reported. There is a subsequent China case-control report for the Gansu Province of China (Wang et al 2002) that shows a positive Odds Ratio above 150 Bq m^{-3} but was not included here. From Figures 16 and 17 of Part II, the mean and maximum and minimum human lung dose responses from combined radon progeny particles and low LET human radiation charged particle traversals are shown.

Research data is emerging in support of abnormal cells as being a key property of carcinogenesis and higher levels of organization such as tissues and organs play an important role. The extensive *in vivo* mice studies (Mitchel et al (1999, 2002, 2003, 2004, Mitchel 2006, 2007a, 2007b, 2008), show that Adaptive Response protection impacts on tumor development and progression. Cancer does not however develop at the tissue or organ level. It is universally accepted that cancers, including lung cancer, starts in a single cell. BEIR VI (1999) acknowledges this. We take the liberty to quote from the "Executive Summary" statement for DOE's Low Dose Radiation Research Program (DOE 1999). The summary begins "Each and every cell in the human body is constantly engaged in a life and death struggle to survive "in spite of itself"." Later in the second paragraph in bold print it states "Thus, a crucial, yet unanswered, question in radiobiology is whether the biological damage induced by low doses and low dose rates of radiation is repaired by the same cellular processes and with the same efficiency as normal oxidative damage that is a way of life for every living cell". Even later in the summary it states "The research program will build on advances in modern molecular biology and instrumentation, not available during the previous 50 years of radiation biology research, to address the effects of very low levels of exposure to ionizing radiation. It will concentrate on understanding the relationship that exists between normal endogenous processes that deal with oxidative damage and processes responsible for the detection and repair of low levels of radiation-induced damage." It is universally understood that the damage inducing carcinogenesis begins solely within the cell, not tissue or organ, although these are impacted by tumor development and metastasis.

This work highlights future research needs. Neither alpha particle Bystander nor low LET Adaptive Response or combined *in vitro* experiments have been conducted, to a

139

reasonable extent, directly with the basal and secretory lung cells. The alpha particle LET and RBE broadbeam *in vitro* experiments of Miller et al (1995) need to be repeated with immortalized basal and secretory cells. Similarly, the low LET Adaptive Response experiments of Dr. Redpaths group need to be repeated with the immortalized basal and secretory cells. Very low doses should be used, below the AR threshold $<z_1>$ values to examine protective Bystander Effect. It is not known if there is a distinction between chromosome damage from Bystander signals and from Direct Damage.

With the hundreds of thousands of mice that have been sacrificed for radon studies, none have involved simultaneous exposure to internal radon progeny alpha lung and external low level low LET radiations, to look for AR, as compared to just internal radon as controls [similar to Dr. Mitchels priming exposures (Mitchel et al 1999, 2002, 2003, 2004, Mitchel 2006, 2007a, 2007b, 2008) examining AR for other biological "endpoints"]. The problem however is that at the higher radon concentrations, such as used by Cross (1988), to accelerate cancer induction in the animals, the doses are in the Direct Damage Region above the Adaptive Response Region and even in the EDE region.

Use of Underground Miners Lung Cancer Risk Data for Domestic and Workplace Radon Levels

The BEIR VI (1999) relies heavily on the lung cancer data from underground miner cohorts. From the work presented here, it would appear that extrapolation from underground miners lung cancer risks (Lubin et al 1995a, 1995b) to lower domestic radon level risks may be fundamentally inappropriate due to the different type cellular damage involved i.e. Bystander Effect Damage at domestic levels and Direct Damage at underground mine levels (See Section 4.2.e of Part I). In Figures 10 and 12 of Part I and the case-control results, it is shown that radon lung cancer induction at human domestic and workplace radon levels is from Bystander lung cell damage. Based on our analysis, only above about 500 Bq m^{-3} of radon is there evidence of Direct Damage induction of human lung cancer from the case-control studies, but this is the primary radon level of exposure for the underground miners. In Figure 10, it is shown that the underground miners were exposed to radon levels where multiple lung cell alpha traversal were prevalent during the 30 day mitotic cycle and thus Direct Damage and a different dose response shaped curve is experienced as evidenced by Figures 10 and 12 of Part I. In fact the depth of the "U" shaped behavior is deeper for the case-control, high risk response,

140

indicating different lung cancer sensitivity for the two regions than predicted by the representative shape curve in Figure 10 of Part I.

Implications Relative to Human Radiation Exposures for the General Public and Radiation Workers

This study has shown that low LET radiation exposures from environmental and man-made sources and normal human activities can induce cancer preventive Adaptive Response radio-protection mechanisms in human lung tissues. These exposures are mostly whole body exposures with doses on the order of fractions of a mGy per cell cycle for most cells within the human body. The LET of the radiations as shown in Tables A1 and A2 of the Appendix A to Part II are such that a significant portion of human cells throughout the body will receive at least one low LET radiation induced charged particle traversal per cycle and thus experience a reduction in potentially carcinogenic spontaneous cellular damage and damage from external radiations, in particular for radiation workers. We have, from Figure 1B here and Table 1 of the nuclear workers study by Cardis et al (2007), examined the dose distributions of the cohorts included in their study.

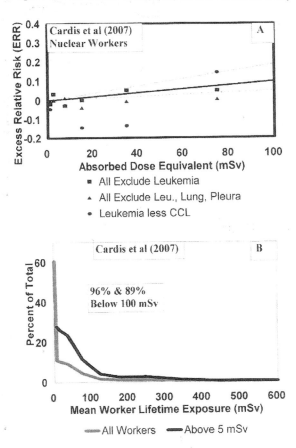

Figure 43 - The Cardis et al (2007) nuclear workers study. Panel A – The low worker dose region showing the Linear No-Threshold Model to be a poor assumption below about 60 mSv. Panel B = Graph of Percent of total workers above the indicated dose showing 96% below 100 mSv and 89% below 100 mSv if the < 5 mSv is neglected.

We reproduce, as Figure 43A, the Cardis et al (2007) data for Excess Relative Risk for cancer from three categories i.e. All Excluding Leukemia, All Excluding Leukemia, Lung and Pleura, and Leukemia less CCL. Below about 70 mSv exposure it is shown that there is either no risk or a negative risk for all three categories. Figure 43B shows that 96% of all workers received a lifetime occupational dose of less than 100 mSv (10 Rem). If we exclude those below 5 mSv, which may be clerical staff that do not enter Radiation Areas, the value is 86%. In our past analysis of Adaptive Response (see Figure 17), we found that the threshold for the Direct Damage component for neoplastic transformation and chromosome aberration production begins at about 10 mGy. An interesting point is that a single alpha particle traversal through a cell delivers more than

10 mSv, thus above the dose where Direct Damage dominates hence would not expect Adaptive Response protection to be observed, as has been the case.

The Ecological Concept for Population Weighting of Radon Radiation Risks

We have shown that ecological and geographical conditions most probably result, in some instances, in a reduction in human lung cancer risks from radon, below the natural occurring zero radon level. We have included all the data in the 23 case-control studies and averaged the cancer risks in the radon exposure range from 0 to 400 Bq m^{-3} has been considered. Although it is conclusive from the high risk data of Krewski et al (2005, 2006) and Darby et al (2005, 2006) that high levels of radon can cause lung cancer it is also evident from the low risk data that a combination of ecological and geological conditions can result in an epidemiological decrease in lung cancers below the spontaneous, zero radon, level for many of the world's populations. Population weighing of the beneficial along with the deleterious aspects of radon may mean radon imposes negligible risk to humans.

A Threshold and Transition Behavior for Initiation of the Direct Damage Region for Alpha Particles

From the application of the composite Microdose Model in Chapter 2 - Part I alpha particle dose response data, it is found that single alpha particle traversals through the cell do not appear to induce neoplastic transformation or chromosome aberrations. The fit of the model demands that there be a threshold and transition involving a second alpha particle traversal through the cell with increasing alpha particle fluence. The idea that more than single hits are necessary to activate the direct damage was first suggested by Miller et al (1999) and here we use the Normal Distribution function simply to empirically shape the dose response curve in the modified Bystander BaD Model. Other causes such as a reduction in the spontaneous damage level by single hits may be the plausible mechanism. The best fit to nine separate data sets in Chapter 2 - Part I found that a Normal Distribution accumulation function with a Mean value of 1.68 traversals and a Standard Deviation of the distribution of 0.62 traversals provides this threshold and transition. Miller et al (1999) first observed this characteristic in comparing single alpha particle microbeam exposures with broadbeam exposures of 10T1/2 fibroblast cells. We have confirmed that multiple traversals are necessary to induce cellular Direct Damage.

Miller et al (1999) commented that this may mean an overestimate of risk at low doses using LNT would occur. We see however that Bystander damage occurs below multiple traversals, at domestic levels, but is, as they note, non-linear and not accurate by LNT extrapolation. We see in the analysis of the case-control studies of Krewski et al (2005, 2006) and Darby et al (2005, 2006) that there is indeed a "U" shaped behavior in their Odds Ratio Lung Cancer Risk curves as determined by our composite Microdose Model analysis and the polynomial best fits in Figures 37 to 40. The analysis of the Miller et al (1999) by Brenner et al (2001) and Little and Wakeford (2001) is inappropriate as shown in Figure 12 since a well-defined Bystander Damage Region would be observed if exposures are performed in that region. This well-defined behavior is clearly seen in Figures 10 and 16 of Chapter 2 - Part I.

Implications with respect to the BEIR VI (1999) and EPA (2003) reports and case- control studies (Darby et al 2005, 2006; Krewski et al 2005, 2006)

The Linear No-Threshold hypothesis was first premised soon after World War II based primarily on the results of studies from the Japanese A-bomb survivors. Nearly every dose response study *a priori* applies the assumption of a linear dose response and it is a natural reaction for the BEIR VI and EPA reports and the case control studies to anticipate a Linear No-Threshold result from their data analysis. BEIR VI does suggest that, based on the new data on the Bystander Effect and Adaptive Response at that time, there may be future evidence that would support a non-linear behavior for radon. Of the 516 pages encompassing BEIR VI, most consists of appendices supporting the conclusions in the Executrive Summary and main report text. Appendix G, containing 61 pages, reports the results of ecological and case-control studies. Figure G-1 provides the dose response data points of 8 case-control studies, that each had more than 200 lung cancer cohorts, that were done before the drafting of BEIR VI. Unlike the Darby et al (2005, 2006) and Krewski et al (2005, 2006) studies shown in Figure 2A and 2B, individual linearized (LNT) graphs of Relative Risks were not provided for each study in BEIR VI (1999).

With the advent of the micro-beam exposure facilities, the effects of single high LET charged particle traversal through single cells were able to be studies primarily at the Columbia University facility (Miller et al 1995, 1999, Zhou et al 2001, Nagasawa and Little 1999, 2002, Hei et al 1999, Sawant et al 2001a, 2001b). From these works, most of which are presented here in Part I, it was conclusively shown that alpha particles traversal

144

through a cell can produce Bystander Damage in adjacent cells. This motivated Drs. Brenner, Little and Sachs to formulate a quantitative Bystander and Direct Damage (BAD) Model for Bystander dose response (Brenner et al 2001). These post-BEIR VI conclusive evidence of the Bystander Effect further resulted in now an *a priori* assumption, by several investigators (Little and Wakeford 2001, Little 2004, Brenner and Sachs 2002, 2003, Brenner et at 2001), that non-linear responsive Bystander Damage in the human lung is the primarily causation on human radon induced lung cancer. The National Research Council's sixth Committee on Biological Effects of Ionizing Radiations (BEIR VI 1999) would be expected now, with this new data which they predicted would come, should embrace a non-linear relative risk from radon. The non-linearity is explicitly demonstrated in Part I in the form of the Representative Alpha Particle Dose Desponse given in Figure 10 of Part I.

What will most likely be vehemently contested in this work herein is the second *a priori* assumption that the Adaptive Response explains the very large variation in the large number of case-control studies encompassing a very, very large number of cohorts. Consulting with a number of peers, no other explanation can be offered for this great variation. As stated above, either the case-control method is totally invalid or there are other mechanisms affecting human lung cancer risks from radon. Several highly respected statistical tests have shown this herein. Thus, the BEIR VI Executive Summary statement "In addition, as discussed in the report, exposure-response relationships estimated from the observational data in miners with low exposures, and from case-control studies of indoor radon, are consistent with linearity." With the overwhelming abundance of very recent new data on the radio-protective effects of Adaptive Response (Azzam et al 1996, Elmore et al 2006, 2006, Ko et al 2004, 2006, Redpath et al 1987, 2001, 2003a, 2003b, Redpath and Antoniono 1998, Shadley and Wiencke 1989, Shadley and Wolff 1987, Shadley et al 1987, Wiencke et al 1986, Wolff et al 1989) and the extensive analysis of Adaptive Response properties and behaviors (Leonard 2005, 2007a, 2007b, 2008a, 2008b, 2008c; Leonard and Leonard 2008), the National Council on Radiation Protection and Measurements (NCRP) have recently accepted the existence of Adaptive Response radio=protection reflected by the *in vitro* research data. Above we point out the value of *in vitro* cell response data, even now, in radio-therapy treatment of human cancer patients. Only recently has Dr. Mitchels group, primarily, [Mitchel et al (1999, 2002, 2003), Mitchel (2006, 2007a, 2007b, 2008)] shown conclusive evidence of

145

Adaptive Response radio-protection in vivo. Other than this work there is little current evidence of Adaptive Response radio-protection in humans from the traversal of single charged particles through human cells.. Many papers have discussed the potential hormesis protective behavior from low doses of ionizing radiations. A classical example, of how human immunity works, is the use of a little flu virus in a flu vaccine to activation human body protection from the flu itself. We have shown that a hormesis protection for human lung cells must occur for human lung cancer risks from radon. There is no reason why low LET background radiation should not provide Adaptive Response radio-protection for other human cells throughout our bodies. We believe that the very recent papers by Dr. John Hart (2011a, 2011b) provides reasonably strong evidence that the small fraction of our annual background radiation from cosmic rays is providing some protection for residents of high elevations in the US. In his first paper (Hart 2011a), he reports that the mortality rate of persons living at average elevations of 559.3 and 2337 feet (above sea level) are 903.3 and 793.8 respectively. In his second paper, Hart (2011b) examines the altitude effect for whites (assuming Caucasian??) and by counties. He shows the average cancer mortality rate of 73.47 ± 18.35 for low elevation counties compared to 53.90 ± 13.76 for high elevation counties. The estimated difference in natural background radiations are 62.5 ± 12.6 mrem and 78.5 ± 2.9 mrem, respectively. This then may provide a second case of human Adaptive Response radio-protection , similar to ours shown herein.

Most of the radio-biology and dosimetry of human lung tissue in the BEIR VI (1999) report and the companion NRC (1991) report are of course valid. The most probable exception is that we premise that high LET Direct Damage is different from high LET Bystander Damage to human lung cells (Ward 1985, 1988, 1995; James et al 2004). Having shown that domestic level radon induced lung cancer is from Bystander Damage and underground miners level radon induced lung cancer is from cell milti-hit Direct Damage, the underground miners data most probably cannot be directly correlated.

146

Chapter 7 - FINAL SUMMARY

This three part study provides perhaps the first direct evidence of Bystander and Adaptive Response effects on humans.

We can tabulate the significant results of the Parts I and II analysis;

1. BEIR VI (1999) and Pooled Case-Control Studies Assumption of Linearity for Human Lung Cancer Risks from Radon

The BEIR VI (1999) assessment of linearity for human lung cancer risks from radon is summarized in their Figure 3-2 and their Executive Summary statement, repeated again here from the Introduction Section as follows: "The choice was to use a linear relationship between risk and low doses of radon progeny without a threshold. The choice was based primarily on considerations related to the stochastic nature of the energy deposition by alpha particles; at low doses, a decrease in dose simply results in a decrease in the number of cells subjected to the same insult. That observation, combined with the evidence that a single alpha particle can cause substantial permanent damage to a cell and that most cancers are of monoclonal origin, provides the mechanistic basis of the use of a linear model at low doses. In addition, as discussed in the report, exposure-response relationships estimated from the observational data in miners with low exposures, and from the case-control studies of indoor radon, are consistent with linearity." The BEIR VI (1999) Figure 3-2 is provided as Figure 1C in the Introduction of Part I. This assumption of linearity of risk is considered basic by the participants in the recent North American (Krewski et al 2005, 2006) and European (Darby et al 2005, 2006) pooled case-control studies with their premise that "The pooling of data from these studies is based on the assumption that between-site differences seen in the observed relationship between lung cancer risk and radon exposure are due to random measurement variability and the true relationship is independent of site locality and only dependent on the carcinogenic sensitivity of human lung tissue to alpha radiation.", which both the Darby et al (2005, 2006) and Krewski et al (2005, 2006) groups assumed to be Linear No-Threshold (LNT) compatible with BEIR VI (1999). We show their linear best fits in Figure 2 of Part I and Figure 1 herein.

2. Analysis of Micro-beam and Broad-beam Alpha Particle *In vitro* Measurements

The micro-beam and broad-beam alpha particle *in vitro* dose response measurements, primarily at the Columbia University accelerator, show that at low radon

147

levels human lung cancers should be from Bystander Damage in human lung tissue (see Figure 10 and 16 of Chapter 2, Part I). Thus the lung cancer Relative Risks dose response should be non-linear according to the Bystander BaD Model and not as premised in Figure 1C. above by BEIR VI (1999) and Figure 2 for Darby et al (2005, 2006) and Krewski et al (2005, 2006).

3. Adaptive Response Radio-protection from Natural Background and Man-made Radiation as the Cause of the Very Large Variation in the Pooled Case-Control Human Lung Cancer Studies

We have noted that low LET induced single charged particle traversals through cells activates Adaptive Response radio-protection against alpha particle chromosome damage and spontaneous cell damage (see Figures 19 of Chapter 3 - Part II). Humans are exposed to low LET radiations from natural background and man-made radiations. Using the UNSCEAR (2000) estimate for these radiations given in Table 1, it is shown in Tables A1, A2 and A3 of Part II – Appendix A, that sufficient lung cell traversals can occur to induce an Adaptive Response reduction in human lung cancer risks. The very large range of the radiations, world-wide, is sufficient to justify the very large variation in lung cancer risks from the case-control studies by a very wide range of AR protections.

4. A Papworth (1975) Poisson Validation Test for Linearity for the Pooled Case-Control Data

In examining the case-control linear best fits in Figure 2, one can only conclude that either 1.) the Odds Ratio method of evaluating lung cancer risk is a very poor method of analysis or 2.) that the above stated premise of "only carcinogenic sensitivity of the human lung" is invalid. For this reason, in Section 3.2 we have applied the Papworth Poisson Validation Test for Linearity (Papworth 1975, Savage and Papworth 2000) to the pooled data with the determination that the data does not reflect a single linear behavior and is over-dispersed when tested for a Poisson distribution about a single linear function – thus reflecting other ancillary influences causing the over-dispersion.

Adaptive Response Radio-Protection as the Only Plausible Ancillary Influence

In Chapter 2, Part I, we have shown that Bystander Damage should be the dominant cause of radon progeny induced human lung cancers at domestic and workplace radon levels. Without any external, ancillary influences, the BEIR VI (1999) and pooled case-control data should indeed reflect a single carcinogenic response, not linearly but

148

following the shape of the Bystander BaD Model illustrated in Figure 3. Morgan (2006) and others have suggested that human response to ionizing radiations should be non-linear and primarily influenced by the Bystander Effect and Adaptive Response radio-protection. The only plausible influence that could cause such a very large range, world-wide, of lung cancer risks from the case-control studies must be AR protection caused by single charged particle traversal through the lung cells e.g. induced from natural background and man-made radiations. Adaptive Response radio-protection is noted in other dose response instances (Redpath and Mitchel 2006, Redpath 2007, Redpath and Elmore 2007).

The Radiation Sources for the Activation of Adaptive Response Protection in Lung Tissue

It is known that Poisson accumulated, low LET radiation induced, single charged particle traversals through the cell nucleus activates the Adaptive Response protective mechanisms. This is found to be independent of the type low LET radiation from X-rays, gamma rays, beta rays, electrons and even high energy protons. Thus all the low LET natural background and man-made radiations, estimated in the United Nations Table 1, will activate Adaptive Response protection. The degree of protection simply depends on the fraction of lung cells receiving charged particle traversals as tabulated in Tables A1, A2 and A3 of the Appendix A. At the UNSCEAR (2000) world-wide average human low LET exposures Table A3 and Figure 32 of Chapter 3 - Part II estimates that a 40% reduction in lung cancer risks occurs at a radon concentration of 400 Bq m^{-3}. At the UNSCEAR (2000) Table 1 minimum and maximum human natural background and man-made radiation levels, it is estimated that 20% and 80% reduction occurs, respectively. Thus, as the pooled case-control studies indicate, a very wide range of human lung cancer risks from radon should be expected world-wide.

Chapter 8 - FINAL CONCLUSIONS

The human lung cancer risk from radon is not linear with increasing radon concentration exposure for two primary reasons. First, the neoplastic transformation frequency and the chromosome aberration rates of cellular damage from alpha particles originates from Bystander Effect damage at normal domestic and workplace radon levels, which has a concave downward response structure with increasing radon. At about 450 Bq m^{-3} concentration, the cellular damage behavior and lung cancer risk experiences a district transition to a quasi-linear-quadratic response with a "U" shaped behavior in this transition region. Second, lung cancer incidence from radon is suppressed by Adaptive Response radio-protection by natural background and man-made low LET radiations routinely experienced by humans. This Adaptive Response protection on a cell-by-cell basis, when experienced in human cells from these whole body exposures, dominates the potential carcinogenic risks from the radon progeny alpha particles. This results in a very large variation in population averaged human lung cancer risks from radon as evidenced by the case-control studies. For human exposures to radon up to about 400 Bq m^{-3} in Europe and North American, and perhaps worldwide depending on geological and ecological conditions, humans have about a 30% chance that there is no lung cancer risk from radon and a 20% chance that the Adaptive Response protection produces a reduced lung cancer risk below the natural, non-radon, spontaneous level. This protection must be afforded to humans with respect to other carcinogens and diseases and should be reflected at the very low annual doses allowed by nuclear workers in the Cardis et al (2007) study (Figures 1B and 43). There is evidence that the cellular sensitive volume for radon induction of lung cancer is the entire cell region (nucleus and cytoplasm) for the basal and secretory cells. Since the dose response is non-linear the RBE for radon progeny alpha particles is not constant.

REFERENCES

Attix FH. 1986, Introduction to radiological physics and radiation dosimetry. John Wiley and Sons, New York, N.Y., USA.

Alavanja MC, Brownson RC, Lubin JH, Berger E, Chang J, and Boice JD. 1994. Residential radon exposure and lung cancer among nonsmoking women. Journal of the National Cancer Institute 86:1829-1837

Alavanja MC, Lubin JH, Mahaffey JA, and Brownson JA. 1999. Residential radon exposure and risk of lung cancer in Missouri. American Journal of Public Health 89:1042-1048

Astrakianakis G, Seixas NS, Ray R, Camp JE, Gao DL, Feng Z, Li W, Wernli KJ, Fitzgibbons ED, Thomas DB, and Checkoway H. 2007. Lung cancer risk among female textile vworkers exposed to endotoxin. Journal of the National Cancer Institute 99:357-364

Azzam SM, DeToledo GP, Raaphorst GP, and Mitchell RE. 1996. Low-dose ionizing radiation decreases the frequency of neoplastic transformation to a low level below the spontaneous rate in C3H 10T1/2 Cells. Radiation Research 146:369-373

Barros-Dios JM, Barreir MA, Ruano-Ravina A, and Figueiras A. 2002. Exposure to residential radon in Spain: a population-based case-control study. American Journal of Epidemiology 156:548-555

BC. 2008. Doses from natural and man made radioactivity - RPS. British Columbia Center for Disease Control. internet web site..

BEAR I 1956. National Research Council, Biological Effects of Atomic Radiation. National Academy Press, Washington, DC

BEIR III 1980. National Research Council, The Effects on Populations of Exposure to Low Levels of Ionizing Radiation. National Academy Press. Washington, DC

BEIR IV 1988. National Research Council, Health Effects of Radon and Other Internally Deposited Alpha-Emitters. National Academy Press. Washington, DC

BEIR V 1990. National Research Council, Health Effects of Exposure to Low Levels of Ionizing Radiation. National Academy Press. Washington, DC

BEIR VI 1999. National Research Council, Health Effects of Exposure to Radon. National Academy Press. Washington, DC

BEIR VII 2006. National Research Council, Health Effects of Exposure to Low Levels of Ionizing Radiation, BEIR VII Phase 2. National Academy Press. Washington, DC

Belyakov OV, Mitchell SA, Parikh D, Randers-Pehrson G, Marino SA, Amundson SA, Geard CR, and Brenner DJ. 2005. Biological effects in unirradiated human tissue induced by radiation damage up to 1 mm away. Proc. Natl. Acad. Sci.102:14203-14208

Blot WJ, Xu Zhoa-Yi, Boice JD, Zhoa D, Stone BJ, Sun J, and Fraumeni JF. 1990. Indoor radon and lung cancer in China. Journal of the National Cancer Institute 82:1025-1030

Bond VP, Varma NN, Sondhaus CA, and Feinendegen LE. 1985. An alternative to absorbed dose, quality, and RBE at low exposures. Radiation Research, Supplement 8:552-557

Brenner DJ. 1997. Review Article. Radiation biology in brachytherapy. Journal of Surgical Oncology 65:66-70.

Brenner DJ, and Hall EJ. 1991. Conditions for the equivalence of continuous to pulsed low dose rate brachytherapy. International Journal of Radiation Oncology Biology and Physics 20:181-190.

Brenner DJ, Little JB, and Sachs RK. 2001, The Bystander Effect in radiation oncogenesis. II. A quantitative model. Radiation Research 155:102-108

Brenner DJ, Martinez AA, Edmundson GK, Mitchell C, Thames HD, and Armour EP. 2002. Direct evidence that prostate tumors show high sensitivity to fractionation (low alpha/beta ratio), similar to late-responding normal tissue. International Journal of Radiation Oncology Biology and Physics 52:6-13.

Brenner DJ, and Sachs RK. 2002. Do low dose-rate Bystander Effect influence domestic radon risks? International Journal of Radiation Biology. 78:593-604

Brenner DJ, and Sachs RK. 2003. Domestic radon risks may be dominated by Bystander Effect – but the risks are unlikely to be greater than we thought. Health Physics Journal 85:103-108

Brooks AL, Khan MA, Duncan A, Buschbom RL, Jostes RF, and Cross RT. 1994. Effectiveness of radon relative to 60Co gamma-rays for induction of micronuclei *in vitro* and in vivo. International Journal of Radiation Biology 66:801-808

152

Brooks AL, Bao S, Harwood PW, Wood BH, Chrisler WB, Khan MA, Gies RA, and Cross FT. 1997. Induction of micronuclei in respiratory tract following radon inhalation. International Journal of Radiation Biology 72:485-495

Cardis E, Vrijheld M, Blettner M, Gilbert E, Hakama M. Hill C, Howe G, Kaldor J, Muirhead CR, Schubauer-Berigan M, Yoshimura T, Bermann F, Cowper G, Fix J, Hacker C, Heinmiller B, Marshall M, Thiery-Chef I, Utterback D, Ahn Y-O, Amoros E, Ashmore P, Auvinen A, Bae J-M, Bernar J, Baiu A, Combalot E, Deboodt P, Diez Sacristan A, Eklof M, Engels H, Engholm G, Gulis G, Habib RR, Holan K, Hyvonen H, Kerekes A, Kurtinaitis J, Malker H, Martuzzi M, Mastauakas A, Monnet A, Moser M, Pearce MS, Richardson DB, Rodriguez-Artalejo FR, Rogel A, Tardy H, Telle-Lamberton, Turai I, Usel M, and Veress K. 2007. The 15-country collaborative study of cancer risk among radiation workers in the nuclear industry: Estimates of radiation related cancer risks. Radiation Research 167:396-416

Carlson DJ, Stewart RD, Jennings XAK, Wang JZ, and Guerrero M. 2004. Comparison of *in vitro* and *in vivo* α / β ratios for prostate cancer. Physical Medical Biolology 49:4477-4491.

Cassoni AM, McMillan TJ, Peacock JH, and Steel GG. 1992. Differences in the level of DNA double-strand breaks in human tumour cell lines following low dose-rate irradiation. European Journal of Cancer 28A:1610-1614.

Cohen BL 1997. Lung cancer risk vs mean radon levels in US counties of various characteristics. Health Physics Journal 72:114-119

Clouvas A, Xanthos S, and Antonopoulos-Domis M. 2001. Extended survey of indoor and outdoor terrestrial gamma radiation in Greek urban areas by in situ gamma spectrometry with a portable Ge detector. Radiation Protection Dosimetry, 94:233-246

Clouvas A, Xanthos S, and Antonopoulos-Domis M. 2003. A combination study of indoor radon and in situ gamma spectrometry measurements in Greek dwellings. Radiation Protection Dosimetry 103:363-366

Clouvas A, Xanthos S, and Antonopoulos-Domis M. 2006. Simultaneous measurements of indoor radon, radon-thoron progeny and high-resolution gamma spectrometry in Greek dwellings. Radiation Protection Dosimetry.

Cross FT. 1988. Radon inhalation studies in animals. US Department of Energy, Pacific Northwest Laboratory; DOE/ER-0396. Washington DC

Curtis S. 1986. Lethal and potentially lethal lesions induced by radiation - a unified repair model. Radiation Research, 106: 252-270.

Clouvas A, Xanthos S, and Antonopoulos-Domis M. 2001. Extended survey of indoor and outdoor terrestrial gamma radiation in Greek urban areas by in situ gamma spectrometry with a portable Ge detector. Radiation Protection Dosimetry, 94:233-246

Darby S, Hill D, Barros-Dios JM, Baysson H, Deo H, Falk R, Hakama M, Kreienbrock L, Kreuzer M, Makelainen I, Muirhead C, Oberaigner, Pershagen G, Ruano-Ravina, Ruosteenoja E, Schaffer A, Tirmarche M, Tomasek L, Wichmann H-E, and Doll R. 2005. Radon in homes and risk of lung cancer: collaborative analysis of data from 13 European case-control studies. Bmj Publishing Group Ltd. 330:223-235.

Darby S, Hill D, Deo H, Auvinen A, Miguel Barros-Dios J, Baysson H, Bochicchio F, Falk R, Farchi S, Figueriras A, Hakama M, Heid I, Hunter N, Kreienbrock L, Kreuzer M, Lagarde F, Makelainen I, Muirhead C, Oberaigner W, Pershagen G, Ruosteenoja E, Schaffrath Rosario A, Tirmarche M, Tomasek L, Whitney E, Wichmann H-E, and Doll R. 2006. Residential radon and lung cancer – detailed results of a collaborative analysis of individual data on 7148 persons with lung cancer and 14208 persons without lung cancer from 13 epidemiologic studies in Europe. Scandinavian Journal of Work and Environmental Health 32: suppli. 1: 1-84.

Day TK, Zeng G, Hooker AM, Bhat M, Scott BR, Turner DR, and Sykes PJ. 2006. Extremely low priming doses of X radiation induce an Adaptive Response for chromosomal inversions in the pKZ1 mouse prostate. Radiation Research 166:757-766

Dasu A, and Denekamp J. 2000, Inducible repair and intrinsic radiosensitivity: a complex   but predictable relationship? Radiation Research, 153: 279-288.

Dey S, Spring PM, Arnold S, Valentino J, Chendil D, Regine WF, Mohiuddin M, and Ahmed MM. 2003. Low-dose fractionation potentiates the effects of paclitaxel in wild-type and mutant p53 head and neck tumor lin

DOE 1999. Low Dose Radiation Research Program, Original Research Program Plan. U. S. Department of Energy Office of Biological and Environmental Research. Washington, D. C. USA

DOE, 2002. Aerial Measuring System Technical Integration Annual Report 2002, National Nuclear Security Administration Nevada Site Office, US Department of Energy, DOE/NV/11718—778. Las Vegas, NV, USA

Duval JS, Jones WJ, Riggle FR, and Pitkin JA. 1989. Equivalent uranium map of the conterminous United States. U. S. Geological Survey Open-File Report 89-478.

Edwards AA, Lloyd DC, and Purrot RJ. 1979. Radiation induced chromosome aberrations and the Poisson distribution. Radiation and Environmental Biophysics 16:89-100

Elmore E, Lao X-Y, Rightnar S, and Redpath JL. 2005. Neoplastic transformation i9n vitro induced by low doses of 232 MeV protons. International Journal of Radiation Biology. 81:291-297

Elmore E, Lao X-Y., Kapadia R, and Redpath JL. 2006. The effect of dose rate on radiation-induced neoplastic transformation *in vitro* by low doses of low-LET radiation. Radiation Research. 166:832-838

Elmore E, Lao X-Y, Kapadia R, Giedzinski E, Limoli C, and Redpath JL. 2008. Low doses of very low-dose-rate low LET radiation suppress radiation-induced neoplastic transformation *in vitro* and induce an adaptive response. Radiation Research 169:311-318

Ellett WH, and Braby LA, 1972. The microdosimetry of 250 kVp and 65 kVp x rays, Co^{60} gamma rays and tritium beta particles. Radiation Research 51:229-243

Enns EG, and Ehler PF. 1993. Notes on random chords in convex bodies. Journal of Applied Probability. 30:889-897

EPA 2003. EPA assessment of risks from radon in homes. EPA 402-R-03-003.United States Environmental Protection Agency. Washington, DC

Feinendegen L, Polycove M, Neumann R. Low-dose cancer risk modeling must recognize up-regulation of protection. Dose-Response Journal 8:227-252.

Folkard M, Vojnovic B, Prise KM, Bowery AG, Locke RJ, Schettino G, and Michael BD. 1997. A charged-particle microbeam, I. Development of an experimental nsystem for targeting cells individually with counted particles. International Journal of Radiation Biology 72:375-385

Furre M, Koritzinsky DR, Olsen A, and Pettersen EO. 1999, Inverse dose-rate effect due to pre-mitotic accumulation during continuous low dose-rate irradiation of cervix carcinoma cells. International Journal of Radiation Biology 75:699-707.

Hall, E.J., 2000, Radiobiology for the Radiologist, Lippincott Williams & Wilkins, New York, NY, USA.

Hall EJ. 2003. The Bystander effect. Health Physics Journal 85:31-35

Harney J, Shah N, Short S, Daley F, Groom N, Wilson GD, Joiner MC, and Saunders MI. 2004a. The evaluation of low dose hyper-radiosensitivity in normal human skin. Radiotherapy Oncology 70:319-329.

Harney J, Short S, Shah N, Joiner MC, and Saunders MI. 2004b. Low dose hyper-radiosensitivity in metastatic tumors. International Journal of Radiation Oncology Biology and Physics 59:1190-1195.

Hart J. 2011a, Cancer mortality in six lowest versus six highest elevation jurisdictions in the U.S. Dose-Response Journal 9:50-58.

Hart J. 2011b, Cancer mortality for a single race in low versus high elevation counties in the U.S. Dose-Response Journal 9:348-355.

HPS 2004. Radiation Risk in Perspective PS010-1, Health Physics Society, Bethesda, MD USA.

Hei TK, Wu LJ, Liu XZ, Vannais D, Waldren CA, and Randers-Pehrson G. 1999, Mutagenic effects of a single and an exact number of ∝ particles in mammalian cells, Proceedings of the National Academy of Science. USA 94:3765-3770

Henderson V, and Enterline PE. 1973. An unusual mortality experience in cotton textile workers. Journal of Ocupational Medicine 15:717-719

Hooker AM, Bhat M, Day TK, Lane JM, Swinburne SJ, Morley AA,, and Sykes PJ. 2004. The linear no-threshold model does not hold for low-dose ionizing radiation. Radiation Research 162:447-452

Huo L, Nagasawa H, and Little JB. 2001. HPRT mutants induced in Bystander cells by very low fluences of alpha particles result primarily from point mutations. Radiation Research 156:521-525

IAEA 2001. Cytogenetic analysis for radiation dose assessment. Technical Series No. 405. International Atomic Energy Agency, Vienna, Austria.

ICRP 1994. Human respiratory tract model for radiological protection. Oxford: Pergamon Press. International Commission on Radiation Protection Report 66, Annals 24 (1-3). London, United Kingdom

ICRP 2004. International Commission on Radiation Protection and Measurements. ICRP Draft report of committee I / Task group, Low dose extrapolation of radiation related cancer risk. London, United Kingdom

ICRU, 1983. International Commission on Radiation Units and Measurements. Microdosimetry, ICRU Report 36, Bethesda, Maryland, USA

Ina Y, and Sakai K. 2005. Further study of prolongation if life span associated with immunological modification by chronic low-dose-rate birradiation in MRL-lpr/lpr mice: Effects of whole-life irradiation. Radiation Research 163:418-423

Iyer R, and Lehnert BE. 2002. Alpha-particle-induced increases in the radioresistance of normal human Bystander cells. Radiation Research 157:3-7

James AC, Birchall A, and Akahani G. 2004. Compararive dosimetry of BEIR VI re-visited. Radiation Protection Dosimetry 108:3-26

Jenkins-Smith H. 2008. Beliefs about radiation: Scientists, the public, and public policy. In: NRCP 2008 Annual Meeting Program, Bethesda, MD page 23.

Joiner MC, Marples B, Lambin P, and Short SC, Turesson I. 2001, Low-dose hypersensitivity: current status and possible mechanisms. International Journal of Radiation Oncology, Biology and Physics 49:379-389

Jones B, Dale RG, Deehan C, Hopkins KI, and Morgan DA. 2001. The role of Biologically effective dose (BED) in clinical oncology. Clinical Oncology (R Coll Radiol) 13:71-81.

Jostes RF, Hul TE, James AC, Cross FT, Schwartz JI, Rotmensch J, Archer RW, Evans HH, Menci J, Bakale G, Rad PS. 1991. *In vitro* exposure of mammalian cells to radon: dosimetric considerations, Radiation Research. 127:211-219

Jostes RF, Hui TE, and Cross FT. 1993. Use of single-cell gel technique to support hit probability calculations in mammalian cells exposed to radon and radon progeny. Health Physics 64:675-679

Jostes RF, Fleck EW, and Morgan TL. 1994. Southern and OCR analysis of HPRT mutations by radon and its progeny. Radiation Research 137:371-384

Kelland LR, Steel GG. 1986. Dose-rate effects in the radiation response of four human tumour xenographs. Radiother Oncol. 7:259-268.

Kellerer AM. 1984, Chord-length distributions and related quantities for spheroids, Radiation Research, 98:425-437

Kellerer AM, and Rossi HH. 1972. The theory of dual radiation action. In: *Current Topics in Radiation Research Quarterly*, Editors M. Ebert and A. Howard, Index Medicus, North-Holland Publishers, Amsterdam, The Netherlands, 8:85-158

Kendal GM. and Smith TJ. 2002. Dose to organs and tissues from radon and its decay products. Journal of Radiological Protection. 22:389-406

Klokov DY, Zaichkina SI, Rozanova OM, Aptikaeva GF, Akhmadieva AK, Smirnova EN, and Balakin VY. 2000. The duration of radioAdaptive Response in mouse bone marrow in vivo. In: Yamada T. et al editors. Biological Effects of Low Dose Radiation. Elsevier Science B.V. Amstrerdam, The Netherlands: pp. 87-91.

Ko SJ, Liao X-Y, Molloi S, Elmore E, and Redpath JL. 2004. Neoplastic transformation *in vitro* after exposure to low doses of mammographic-energy X rays: Qualitative and mechanistic aspects. Radiation Research, 162:646-654

Krewski D, Lubin JH, Zielinski JM, Alavanja M, Catalan VS, Field RW, Klotz JB, Letourneau EG, Lynch CF, Lyon JL, Sandler DP, Schoenberg JB, Steck DJ, Stolwijk JA, Weinberg C, and Wilcox HB. 2005. Residential radon and risk of lung cancer: a combined analysis of 7 North American case-control studies. Epidemiology. 16:137-145

Krewski D, Lubin JH, Zienski JM, Alavanja M, Catalan VS, Field RW, Klotz JB, Letourneau EG, Lynch CF, Lyon JL, Sandler DP, Schoenberg JB, Steck DJ, Stolwijk JA, Weinberg C, and Wilcox HB. 2006. A combined analysis of North American case-control studies of residential radon and lung cancer. Journal of Toxicology and Environmental Health, Part A. 69:533-597

Leonard BE. 1996. High ^{222}Rn levels, enhanced surface deposition, increased diffusion coefficient, humidity, and air change effects. Health Physics 70:372-387

Leonard BE. 2000, Repair of multiple break chromosomal damage -- its impact on the use of the linear-quadratic model for low dose and dose rates. In: The Effects of Low and Very Low Doses of Ionizing Radiation on Human Health, pp 449-462. University of Versailles, Elsevier Science B.V. Amsterdam, The Netherlands

Leonard BE. 2005, Adaptive Response by single cell radiation hits - Implications for nuclear workers, Radiation Protection Dosimetry. 116:387-391

Leonard BE. 2007a, Adaptive Response and human risks: Part I - A microdosimetry dose dependent model, International Journal of Radiation Biology. 83:115-131

Leonard BE. 2007b, Adaptive response: Part II - Modeling for dose rate and time influences, International Journal of Radiation Biology, 83:395-409

Leonard BE. 2007c. Examination of underground miner data for radon progeny size reduction as cause of high radon "inverse" dose rate effect. Health Physic Journal, 93:133-150

Leonard BE. 2007d. Thresholds and transitions for activation of cellular radioprotective3 mechanisms = correlations between HRS/IRR and the "inverse" dose rate effect. International Journal of Radiation Biology, 83:479-489

Leonard BE. 2008a. A composite microdose Adaptive Response (AR) and Bystander Effect (BE) model – application to low LET and high LET data. International Journal of Radiation Biology, 84:681-701

Leonard BE. 2008b. A review: Development of a Microdose Model for analysis of Adaptive Response and Bystander dose response behavior. Dose-Response Journal, 6:115-183

Leonard BE, and Leonard VF. 2008. Mammogram and diagnostic X-rays – evidence of protective Bystander, Adaptive Response (AR) radio-protection and AR retention at high dose. International Journal of Radiation Biology, 84:885-899

Leonard BE. 2009. The range of the Bystander Effect signal in 3-dimensional tissue and estimation of the range in human lung tissue at low radon levels, Radiation Research Journal 171:374-378

Leonard BE, and Lucas AC. 2008. The correlation of hypersensitivity for HRS/IRR and the "inverse" dose rate effect – its potential influence on LDR brachytherapy – A Review. International Journal of Low Radiation. 5:310-355

Leonard BE, and Lucas AC. 2009. LDR brachytherapy – can low dose rate hypersensitivity from the "inverse" dose rate effect cause excessive cell killing to peripherial connective tissues and organs? British Journal of Radiology 82:131-139

Leonard BE, Thompson RE and Beecher GC. 2011a. Human lung cancer risks from radon – Part I – Influence from Bystander Effect – A microdose analysis. Dose-Response Journal, 9:243-292.

Leonard BE, Thompson RE and Beecher GC. 2011b. Human lung cancer risks from radon – Part II – Influence from combined Adaptive Response and Bystander Effect – A microdose analysis. Dose-Response Journal, 9:502-553.

Leonard BE, Thompson RE and Beecher GC. 2012. Human lung cancer risks from radon – Part III – Evidence of influence of combined Bystander and Adaptive Response effects on radon case-control studies – A microdose analysis. Dose-Response Journal, In Press.

Levin LI, Gao YT, Blot WJ, Zheng W, and Fraumeni JF Jr. 1987. Decreased risk of lung cancer in the cotton textile industry of Shanghai. Cancer Research 47:5777-5781

Little MP, and Wakeford R. 2001. The Bystander Effect in C3H 10T1/2 cells and radon induced lung cancer. Radiation Research, 156:695-699

Little MP. 2004. The Bystander Effect model of Brenner and Sachs fitted to lung cancer data in 11 cohorts of underground miners, and equivalence of fit oa a linear relative risk model with adjustment for attained age and age at exposure. Journal of Radiological Protection. 24:243-255

Llorca J, Bringas-Bollada M, and Quindos-Poncela LS. 2007. No evidence of a link between household radon concentrations and lung cancer in Cantabria, Spain. Archivos de Bronconeumologia. 43: 696.

Lloyd DC, Edwards AA, Leonard A, Deknudt GL, Natajan AT, Obe G, Palitti F, Tanzarella C, Tawn EJ. 1988. Frequencies of chromosome aberrations induced in human blood lymphocytes by low doses of X-rays. International Journal of Radiation Biology 53:49-55

Lubin JH, Boice JD Jr, Edling C, Hornung RW, Howe G, Kunz E, Kusiak RA, Morrison HI, Radford EP, Samet JM, Tirmarche M, Woodward A, Yao, SX, Pierce DA. 1995a. Lung cancer in radon-exposed miners and estimation of risk from indoor exposure. Journal of the National Cancer Institute 87:817-827

Lubin JH, Boice Jr. JD, Edling C, Hornung RW, Howe G, Kunz E, Kusiak RA, Morrison HI, Radford EP, Samet JM, Tirmarche M, Woodward A, and Yao, SX. 1995b. Radon Exposed Underground Miners and Inverse Dose-Rate (Protraction Enhancement) Effects. Health Phys. 69:494-500

Makelainen I, Arvela H, and Voutilainen A. 2001. Correlations between radon concentration and indoor gamma dose rate, soil permeability and dwelling substructure and ventilation. The Science and Total Environment. 272:283-289

McMillan TJ, Eady JJ, Holmes A, Peacock JH, and Steel GG. 1989, The radiosentivity of human neuroblastoma: A cellular and molecular study. International Journal of Radiation Biology. 56:651-656.

Marples B, Wouters BG, Collis SJ, Chambers AJ, and Joiner MC. 2004. A Review - Low-dose hyper-radiosensitivity: A consequence of ineffective cell cycle arrest of radiation- damaged G_2-phase cells. Radiation Research 161:247-255.

Martin SG, Miller RC, Geard CR, and Hall EJ. 1995. The biological effectiveness of radon-progeny alpha particles. IV. Morphological transformation of Syrian hamster embryo cells at low doses. Radiation Research 142:70-77

Metting N, Kofhler A, Nagasawa H, John M and Jo C. 1995. Design of a benchtop alpha particle irradiator. Health Physics Journal 68:627-730.

Miller RC, Marino SA, Brenner DJ, Martin SG, Richards M, Randers-Pehrson G, and Hall EJ. 1995. The biological effectiveness of radon-progeny alpha particles. II. Oncogenic transformation as a function of linear energy transfer. Radiation Research, 142:54-60

Miller RC, Randers-Pehrson G, Geard CR, Hall EJ, and Brenner DJ. 1999, The oncogenic transforming potential of the passage of single α particles through mammalian cell nuclei. Proceedings of the National Academy of Science 96:19-22

Mitchel, R.E.J., Jackson, J.S., McCann, R.A. and Borcham, D.R. 1999. Adaptive Response modification of latency for radiation-induced mycloid leukemia in CBA/H mice. Radiation Research 152: 273-279

Mitchel REJ, Dolling J-A, Misonoh J, and Boreham DR. 2002. Influence of prior exposure tom low-dose adapting radiation on radiation-induced teratogenic effects in fetal mice with varying Trp-53 function. Radiation Research 158:458-463

Mitchel REJ. 2006. Low doses of radiation are protective *in vitro* and in vivo. Evolutionary origins. Dose-Response Journal 4:75-90

Mitchel REJ. 2007a. Cancer and low dose responses in vivo: Implications for radiation protection. Dose-Response Journal. 5:284-291

Mitchel, REJ. 2007b. Low doses of radiation reduce risk in vivo. Dose-Response Journal 5:1-10

Mitchel REJ, Jackson JS, Morrison DP, and Carlise SM. 2003. Low doses of radiation increase the latency of spontaneous lymphomas and spinal ostcosarcomas in cancer prone, radiation sensitive Trp53 heterozygous mice. Radiation Research 159:320-327

Mitchel REJ. 2008. A lower dose threshold for the *in vivo* protective Adaptive Response to radiation. Tumorigenesis in chronically exposed normal and Trp-53 heterozygous C57BL/6 mice. Radiation Research 170:765-775

Mitchel REJ. 2010. The dose window for radiation induced protective adaptive response Dose-Response Journal 8:192-208.

Mitchell SA, Marino SA, Brenner DJ, and Hall EJ. 2004. Bystander Effect and Adaptive Response in C3H 10T1/2 cells. International Journal of Radiation Biology 80:465-472

Morgan WF. 2003a. Non-targeted and delayed effects of exposure to ionizing radiation: I, Radiaion-induced genomic instability and Bystander Effect *in vitro*. Radiation Research 159:567-580

Morgan WF. 2003b. Non-targeted and delayed effects of exposure to ionizing radiation: I, Radiaion-induced genomic instability and Bystander Effect *in vivo*. Radiation Research 159:581-596

Morgan WF. 2006. Will radiation-induced Bystander Effect or adaptive responses impact on the shape of the dose response relationships at low doses of ionizing radiation? Dose-Response. 4:257-262

Mothersill C, and Seymour CB. 1997. Medium from irradiated human epithelial cells but not human fibroblasts reduces the clonogenic survival of unirradiated cells. International Journal of Radiation Biology, 71:421-427

Mothersill C, and Seymour C. 2005. Radiation-induced Bystander Effect: are they good, bad or both? Medicine, Conflict and Survival. 21:101-110

Nagasawa H, and Little JB. 1999. Unexpected sensitivity to the induction of mutations by very low doses of alpha-particle radiation: Evidence of a Bystander effect. Radiat. Res. 152:552-557

Nagasawa H, and Little JB. 2002. Bystander Effect for chromosome aberrations induced in wild-type and repair deficient CHO cells by low fluences of alpha particles. Mutation Research. 508:121-129

Nagasawa H, Huo I, and Little JB. 2003. Increased Bystander mutagenic effect in DNA double-strand break repair-deficient mammalian cells. International Journal of Radiation Biology, 79:35-41

Nelson JM, Brooks AL, Metting NF, Khan MA, Buschbom RL, Duncan A, Miick R, and Braby LA. 1996. Clastogenic effects of defined numbers of 3.2 MeV alpha particles on individual CHO-K1 cells. Radiation Research 145:568-574

Nikezic D, and Yu KN. 2001. Alpha hit frequency due to radon decay products in human lung cells. International Journal of Radiation Biology, 77:559-565

NOAA 2008. Physics of the airborne gamma SWE measurement. National Operational Hydrologic Remote Sensing Center, National Weather Service, NOAA, Washington, DC

NRC 1991. Comparative dosimetry of Radon in mines and homes. National Research Council, National Academy of Science, Washington, DC

162

Papworth D. 1975. Curve fitting by maximum likelihood. Radiation Botany 15:127-131

Pilkyte L, and Butkus D., 2005. Influence of gamma radiation of indoor radon decay products on absorbed dose rate. Journal of Environmental Engineering and Landscape Management. XIII:65-72

Pohl-Ruling J.1988, Chromosome aberrations in man in areas with elevated natural radioactivity. In: Bezelius Symposium XV :103-111

Pohl-Ruling J. 1992. Low level dose induced chromosome aberrations in human blood lymphocytes. Radiation Protection Dosimetry 43:623-627

Porstendorfer J. 2001. Physical Parameters and Dose Factors of the Radon and Thoron Decay Products. Radiation Protection Dosimetry 94:365-373

Preston DL, Ron E, Tokuoka S, Funanmoto S, Nishi N, Soda M, Mabuchi K, and Kodama K. 2007. Solid cancer incidence in atomic bomb survivors. Radiation Research 168:1-64

Randers-Pehrson G, Geard CR, Johnson G, Elliston CD, and Brenner DJ. 2001. The Columbia University single-ion microbeam. Radiation Research. 156:210-214

Redpath JL, and Antoniono RJ. 1998. Induction of an Adaptive Response against low dose gamma radiation. Radiation Research 149:517-520

Redpath JL, Liang D, Taylor TH, Cristie C, and Elmore E. 2001. The shape of the dose-response curve for radiation-induced neoplastic transformation In Vitro: Evidence for an Adaptive Response against neoplastic transformation at low doses of low-LET radiation. Radiation Research. 156:700-707

Redpath JL, Lu Q, Lao X, Molloi S, and Elmore E. 2003. Low doses of diagnostic X-rays protect against neoplastic transformation in vitro. International Journal of Radiation Biology 79:235-240.

Redpath JL, and Mitchel REJ. 2006. Letter to Editor: Enhanced biological effectiveness of low energy X-rays and implications for the UK breast screening programme. British Journal of Radiology. 79:854-855

Redpath, J.L. 2007. Health risks of low photon energy imaging. Radiation Protection Dosimetry, 122, 528-533.

Redpath JL, and Elmore E. 2007. Radiation-induced neoplastic transformation in vitro, hormesis and risk assessment, Dose-Response Journal 5:123-130

Rockwell T III. 1956. Reactor Shielding Design Manual. U. S. Atomic Energy Commission. McGraw-Hill, New York.

Rossi HH, and Zaider M. 1997. Radiogenic lung cancer, the effects of low doses of low linear energy transfer (LET) radiation. Radiation and Environmental Biophysics. 36/2:85-88.

Rossi HH. 1999. Risks from less than 1.0 milliseverts. Radiation Protection Dosimetry. 83:277-279

Savage JRK, and Papworth DG. 2000. Constructing a 2B calibration curve for retrospecrive dose reconstruction. Radiation Protection Dosimetry 88:69-76

Sawant SG, Randers-Pehrson G, Geard CR, Brenner DJ, and Hall EJ. 2001a. The Bystander Effect in radiation oncogenesis: I. Transformation in C3H 10T1/2 cells *in vitro* can be initiated in the unirradiated neighbors of irradiated cells. Radiation Research 155:397-401

Sawant SG, Randers-Pehrson G, Metting NF, and Hall EJ., 2001b, Adaptive Response and Bystander Effect induced by radiation in C3 10T1/2 cells in culture. Radiation Research, 156:177-180

Schmid E, and Roos H. 2008, Influence of the Bystander phenomenon on the chromosome aberration pattern in human lymphocytes induced by *in vitro* α – particle exposure. Radiation and Environmental Biophysics 48:181-187

Schollinberger H, Mitchel REJ, Crawford-Brow3n DJ, and Hofmann W. 2006. A model for the induction of chromosome aberrations through direct and Bystander mechanisms. Radiation Protection Dosimetry 122:275-281

Schoenberg JB, Klotz JB, Wilcox HB, Nicholls GP, Gil-del-Real MT, Sternhagen A, and Mason TJ. 1990. Case-control study of residential radon and lung cancer among New Jersey women. Cancer Research 50:6520-6524

Schoenberg JB, Klotz JB, Wilcox HB, and Szmaciasz SF. 1992. A case-control study of radon and lung cancer among New Jersy women. Indoor Radon and Lung Cancer: Reality or Myth?, Sponsored by the United States Department of Energy and Battelle Northwest Laboratories, ed. F. T. Cross, pp. 905-918. Battelle Press.Columbus, OH

Schwartz GF, Klingele EK, and Rybach L. 2008. Data processing and mapping in airborne radiometric surveys. Institut fur Geophysik ETHZ, CH-8093. Zurich, Switzerland.

Shadley JK, and Wiencke JK. 1989. Induction of the Adaptive Response by X-rays is dependent on radiation intensity. International Journal of Radiation Biology, 56:107-118

Shadley JH, and Wolff S. 1987. Very low doses of x-rays can cause human lymphocytes to become less susceptible to ionizing radiation, Mutagenesis 2:95-96

Shadley JD, Afzal V, and Wolff S. 1987. Characterization of the Adaptive Response to ionizing radiation induced by low doses of x rays to human lymphocytes. Radiation Research, 111:511-517

Shao C, Folkard M, Michael BD, and Prise KM. 2004. Targeted cytoplasmic irradiation induces Bystander responses. Proceedings of the National Academy of Science. 101:13495-13500

Simmons JA, and Richards SR. 1988. The volumes of rat and human lung cells as measured by an image analyzer. Clinical, Physical and Physiological Measurements 9:363-369

Slonina D, Biesaga B, Urbanski K, and Kojs Z. 2007. Low-dose radiation response of primary keratinocytes and fibroblasts from patients with cervix cancer. Radiation Research 167:251-259.

Steel GG, Deacon JM, Duchesne GM, Horwich A, Kelland LR, and Peacock JH. 1987. Review Article – The dose-rate effect in human tumour cells, 9: 299-310.

Stephens CT, Eady JJ, Peacock JH, and Steel GG. 1987. Split-dose and low dose-rate recovery in four experimental tumour systems. International Journal of Radiation Biology 52:157-170.

Suzuki MH, Geard CR, and Hei TK. 2004. Effect of medium on chromatin damage in Bystander mammalian cells. Radiation Research 162:264-269

Szluinska M, Edwards AA, and Lloyd DC. 2005. Statistical methods for biological dosimetry. Health Protection Agency Report HPA-RPD-011, Centre for Radiation, Chemical and Environmental Hazards, Radiation Protection Division, Chilton, Oxfordshire UK.

Thames HD. 1985, An "incomplete-repair" model for survival after fractionated and continuous irradiations. International Journal of Radiation Biology, 47: 319-339.

Thompson RE, Nelson DF, Popkin JH, and Popkin Z. 2008. Case-control study of lung cancer risk from residential Radon exposure in Worcester County, Massachusets. Health Physics Journal 94:228-241

Tome WA, and Howard SP. 2007. On the possible increase in local tumour control probability for gliomas exhibiting low dose hyper-radiosensitivity using a pulsed schedule. British Journal of Radiology 80:32-37

Tubiana M, Aurengo A, Averbeck D, Bonnin A, Le Guen B, Masse R, Monier R, Valleron AJ, and de Vathaire F. 2005. Dose-effect relationships and the estimation of the carcinogenic effects of low doses of ionizing radiation. Joint Report no. 2, Academie National de Medicine, Institute de France - Academie des Sciences. Paris, France.

Tubiana M, Aurengo A, Averbeck D, and Masse R. 2006. The debate on the use of linear no threshold for assessing the effects of low doses. Journal of Radiation Protection. 26:317-324

Tubiana M, Aurengo A, Averbeck D, and Masse R. 2007. Low-dose risk assessment: Comments on the summary of the international workshop. Radiation Research, 167:742-744

UNSCEAR (United Nations Scientific Committee on the Effects of Atomic Radiation). 2000. Sources and Effects of Ionizing Radiation. UNSCEAR Report to the General Assembly, Volume I: Sources. United Nations. New York, NY USA

Varma NN, Baum JW, Kliauga P, and Bond VP. 1981. Microdosimetric parameters for photons as a function of depth in water using wall-less and walled counters. Radiation Research 88:466-475

Wang GJ, and Cai L. 2000. Induction of cell-proliferation hormesis and cell-survival Adaptive Response in mouse hematopoietic cells by whole-body low-dose radiation. Toxicological Sciences 53:369-376

Wang Z, Lubin J, Wang L, Zhang S, Boice JD Jr, Cui H, Zhang S, Conrath S, Xia Y, Shang B, Brenner A, Lei S, Metayer C, Cao J, Chen KW, Lei S, and Kleinerman RA. 2002. Residential radon and lung cancer risk in a high-exposure area of Gansu Province, China. American Journal of Epidemiology 155:554-564

Ward JF. 1985. Biochemistry of DNA leisions. Radiation Research 104:S-103-S-111

Ward JF. 1988. DNA damage produced by ionizing radiation in mammalian cells; Identies, mechanisms of formation and repairability. Progress in Nucleic Acid Research and Molecular Biology 35:95-124

Ward JF. 1995. Commentary-Radiation Mutagenesis: The initial DNA leisions responsible. Radiation Research 142:362-368

Wiencke JK, Afzal V, Oliveri G, and Wolff S., 1986, Evidence That [^{3}H] Thymidine-induced Adaptive Response of human lymphocytes to subsequent doses of x-ray involves the induction of a chromosomal repair mechanism. Mutagenesis 1:375-380

Wolff S, Wiencke JK, Afzal V, Youngbloom J, and Cortes I. 1989. The Adaptive Response of human lymphocytes to very low doses of ionizing radiation: a case of induced chromosomal repair with induction of specific proteins. In: Low Dose Radiation: Biological Bases of Risk Assessment. K.I. Baverstock and J.W. Stather, Eds. Pp 446-454. Taylor and Francis, London, United Kingdon

Wolff S, Jostes RF, Cross FT, Hui TE, Afzal V, and Wiencke JK. 1991. Adaptive Response of human lymphocytes for the repair of radon-induced chromosomal damage Mutation Research 250:299-306

Wollenberg HA, Revzan KL, and Smith AR. 1994. Application of airborne gamma spectrimetric survey data to estimating terrestrial gamma ray dose rates: an example in California. Health Physics 66:10-16

Zhou H, Suzuki M, Randers-Pehrson G, Vannais D, Chen G, Trosko JE, Waldren CA, and Hei TK. 2001. Radiation risk to low fluences of α particles may be greater than we thought. Proceedings of the National Academy of Science 98:14410-14415

Zhou H, Randers-Pehrson G, Geard CR, Brenner DJ, Hall EJ, and Hei T. 2003. Interaction between radiation-induced Adaptive Response and Bystander mutagenesis in mammalian cells. Radiation Research. 160:512-516

Zhou, H., Randers-Pehrson, G. Waldren, C.A. and Hei TK. 2004. Radiation-induced Bystander Effect and Adaptive Response in mammalian cells. Advances in Space Research. 34, 1368-1372.

APPENDICES

PART II - APPENDIX A

Examination of Potential Adaptive Response Suppression of Radon Alpha Particle Human Lung Cellular Bystander and Direct Damage

A.1 Sources Adaptive Response Producing Low LET Radiations Received by Humans

In Section 3.3.a.1 of Chapter 4 of Chapter 4, Part III above, we note that Americans receive a population averaged annual radiation dose equivalent of about 2.4 mSv of background radiation of which 39 % is low LET, consisting primarily of about 20% terrestrial gamma rays, 12% a cosmic ray component and 7% internal (ingestion) component, and 52 % from high LET Radon progeny (BEIR VII 2006, UNSCEAR 2000). It is also noted that we receive an annual average of about 0.5 mSv of man-made radiation, of which at least 98 % is low LET. Thus, the major components of our total population averaged annual dose of 2.9 mSv is about 1.44 mSv low LET and about 1.25 mSv high LET Radon progeny alphas. We shall use two methods to evaluate the possibility and probability of Adaptive Response radio-protection against the incidence of lung cancer. Adaptive Response has been shown to be activated by Poisson accumulated; low LET radiation produced single charged particle traversals through individual cells. Because the energy deposited to the lung cells per traversal varies with the LET of the charged particles, to estimate the potential of the radiations to induce Adaptive Response reduction in lung cancer risks from radon, we must evaluate each source of radiation. We will first examine the low LET radiations charged particle traversal frequency for the different human exposure sources at the above cited average levels. For consistency we will use the UNSCEAR world-wide average annual doses for each component. Table 1 lists these as given in UNSCEAR (2000). Figure 44 provides the gamma ray specta for terrestrial background radiation and the Uranium, Thorium and Potassium 40 components from NaI spectrometry.

169

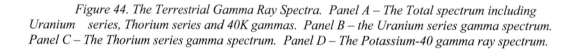

Figure 44. The Terrestrial Gamma Ray Spectra. Panel A – The Total spectrum including Uranium series, Thorium series and 40K gammas. Panel B – the Uranium series gamma spectrum. Panel C – The Thorium series gamma spectrum. Panel D – The Potassium-40 gamma ray spectrum.

Beta Ray Dose From the Radon Progeny

Along with the two radon progeny alpha emissions, there are 14 progeny gamma rays, ranging in energies from 0.05 to 2.44 MeV, and 7 progeny beta particles, ranging in maximum energies from 0.69 to 3.26 MeV.

Figure 44, The Decay Scheme for Radium-226 and its progeny

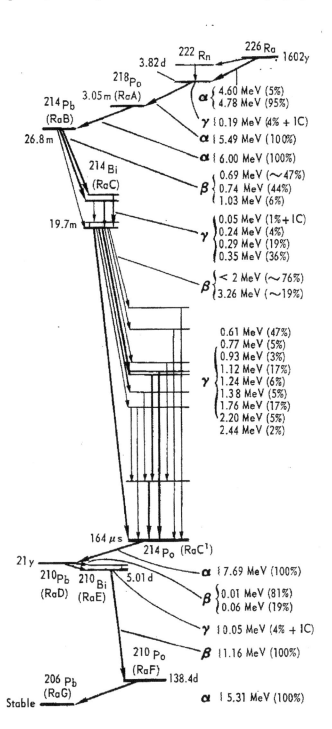

Figure 45 provides the decay scheme for ²²⁶Ra, showing the ²²²Rn and the progeny radiations.

In Table A1, we list the gammas above 1% emission and the 7 beta rays from the Radon progeny.

TABLE A1 – Primary Low LET Internal and External Radiations to Which Human Lungs are Exposed and LET Values

Isotope	Type	Energy (MeV)	Percent of Decays	LET Tissue (keV/um)	Isotope	Type	Energy (MeV)	Percent of Decays	LET Tissue (keV/um)
K-40	Gamma	1.46	11	0.245	Thorium Series				
	Beta+	0.49	11	0.241	Ra-228	Beta	0.055	100	0.610
	Beta-	1.33	89	0.191	Ac-228	Gamma	0.34	15	0.410
						Gamma	0.91	25	0.320
U Series (and Radon Progeny)						Gamma	0.96	20	0.210
Pb-214	Gamma	0.30	19	0.430		Beta	1.18	35	0.195
	Gamma	0.35	36	0.400		Beta	1.75	12	0.186
	Beta	0.65	50	0.227		Beta	2.09	12	0.183
	Beta	0.71	40	0.220	Pb-212	Gamma	0.24	47	0.470
	Beta	0.98	6	0.202		Gamma	0.30	3.2	0.430
Bi-214	Gamma	0.61	47	0.360		Beta	0.35	81	0.296
	Gamma	1.12	17	0.295		Beta	0.59	14	0.234
	Gamma	1.77	17	0.200	Bi-212	Gamma	0.04	2	
	Gamma	2.21	5	0.135		Gamma	0.73	7	0.360
	Gamma	2.45	2	0.080		Gamma	1.62	1.8	0.230
	Beta	1.00	23	0.202		Beta	1.55	5	0.188
	Beta	1.51	40	0.188		Beta	2.26	55	0.183
	Beta	3.26	19	0.187	Tl-208	Gamma	0.51	23	0.400
Po-218	Alpha	6.00	100	100		Gamma	0.58	86	0.375
Po=214	Alpha	7.69	100	80		Gamma	0.86	12	0.325
						Gamma	2.61	100	0.060
Cosmic "Rays"						Beta	1.28	25	0.192
	Proton	200	89	0.4		Beta	1.52	21	0.188
	Helium		11			Beta	1.80	50	0.185

In the radon *in vitro* exposure environment for the Pohl-Ruling human lymphocyte exposures shown in Figure 19D of the main text, these low LET progeny radiations are estimated to deliver only about 5% of the Radon alpha lung dose (Josters et al 1991) if ^{218}Po is deposited within the cell medium since a significant fraction of the betas escape from the *in vitro* cultures with most of their kinetic energies. For human exposure to radon and its airborne progeny, we need to evaluate the indoor equilibrium levels of the progeny. The four decay products are ^{218}Po (alpha emitter, 3.05 minute half-life), ^{214}Pb (beta emitter, 26.8 minute half-life), ^{218}Bi (beta emitter, 19.7 minute half-life) and ^{214}Po (alpha emitter, 164 second half-life). If they were in secular equilibrium the ratio of betas-to-alphas would be 1 to 1. The ratios have been extensively studied (NRC 1991, BEIR VI 1999) and as a rule they are not in equilibrium. The typical ratio for the decay products are 5 (^{218}Po)/ 3 (^{214}Pb) / 2 (^{214}Bi) / 2 (^{214}Po). This gives a beta-to-alpha ratio of 5 to 7. The equilibrium fraction chosen is thus about 0.42. By tabulating the energies of the beta decays and the alpha decays, we compute that if all the kinetic energies are deposited in the lung tissue then the betas deposition will be 24.6 % of the alpha deposition energy. We must consider the fact that the range of the ^{214}Po betas (2.0 and 3.26 MeV) are about 0.98 and 1.63 cm respectively in tissue. These significant ranges, in terms of cell diameters, compared to the *in vitro* exposure samples for the Pohl-Ruling exposures is why the beta dose was only 5% of the alpha dose. The extensive study of the physiology of the lung with respect to alpha particle exposure is given in NRC (1991). The adult lung has a total mass of from 300 to 400 grams. Its volume is about 5.5 liters, so most of the lung consists of conducting airways and blood circulatory system for exchange of carbon dioxide laden old air with oxygen fresh new air. From a geometric viewpoint, the two lung sections, consisting of 150 to 200 grams of tissue and volume of 2.75 liters, will mean that at least 75% of the beta rays energy will be deposited within the lung tissue. Then our best estimate is that the beta dose to the lung from the radon progeny is about $20 \pm 5\%$ of the alpha dose (in Gy) to the lung. These beta rays are thus important in our evaluation of low LET Adaptive Response effects from the Radon progeny and we shall use a lung beta dose of 20% of the Radon alpha dose in our calculations shown in Tables A1 and A2.

Terrestrial Radiations

The properties of terrestrial radiations are well known. They consist of three basic components, Potasium-40, the Uranium natural radioactive series and the Thorium natural radioactive series. There have been extensive United States (US) national and worldwide surveys of these radiations. As Figure 44, we provide the gamma ray spectrum for background radiation as determined with a high resolution Germanium solid-state radiation detector and a multi-channel spectrometer system. Shown is the single 1.461 MeV gamma ray from ^{40}K, the 5 ^{214}Bi gamma rays from the Uranium series and the 3 gamma rays from the Thorium series. As Figures 44B, 44C and 44D, we show the separate resolved spectra for ^{40}K, the Uranium series and the Thorium series gamma rays. Knowing the gamma ray energies and the relative decay fractions, the effective LETs of each radiation component is provided in Table A1. UNSCEAR (2000) estimates the separate annual dose equivalent components to be 0.122 mSv/a, 0.195 mSv/a and 0.183 mSv/a for Uranium, Thorium and Potassium-40, respectively, using the UNSCEAR world-wide annual average terrestrial gamma ray dose equivalent is 0.50 mSv/a. These values are used in Table A2 to compute the Specific Energy Hits per radon 30 day cell cycle.

Cosmic "Rays", Internal and Medical Radiation Exposures

We have put quotation marks around the word <u>ray</u> because the normal cosmic ray spectrum consists primarily of high energy protons (about 89%) and helium atoms (about 10%) - not rays. The kinetic energy of the protons are about 200 MeV. Elmore et al (2005) have measured the dose response of 232 MeV proton exposure to HeLa x skin cells (see Figure 4D herein) showing an AR protection. The LETs used in Table A1 for the photons, beta rays and protons are estimated from Attix (1986), Hall (2000) and Figure 1-1 of ICRP (2006).

UNSCEAR estimates that most of the internal dose for humans to be about 0.180 mSv from ingestion of Potassium-40 in food products. The remaining 0.120 mSv dose equivalent is primarily from the Uranium and Thorium series isotopes. The annual medical exposure of 0.40 mSv/a is broken down into various world population with respect to health care capabilities. The exposures are primarily from low energy diagnostic X-rays, mammograms, CT scans and some internal medicine isotopic injects as tracers.

Computations in Tables A1 and A2 for Low LET Charged Particle Traversals from UNSCEAR Annual Doses

We have explained the data in Table A1 in the previous section. The Equation (7) in Chapter 2 – Part I of the main text was used to compute the mean Specific Energy depositions per radiation induced charged particle traversal (hit) in units of cGy per hit. In Table A2, we have computed the Specific Energy depositions per hit (traversal) in Columns 4 and 5. This was based on the LETs of the radiation and the lung cell total and nucleus diameters (Columns 2 and 3) for the bronchial basal, bronchial secretory and bronchiolar secretory sensitive lung cells.

TABLE A2 - **Values of Parameters Used to Compute Estimated Charged Particle Traversals (Specific Energy Hits) to the Human Lung from Low LET Terestrial, Internal, Medical and Cosmic Radiations Including Cosmic High Energy Protons. Also, Lung Deposited Radon Progeny Low LET Beta Radiations.**

Component	LET (keV/um)	Cell Diameter Cell (um)	Nucleus (um)	$<z_1>$ (cGy/Hit) Cell	Nucleus	Dose Rates Radon 7.0 nGy/hBqm-3 Terrestrial 0.50mSv/a Cosmic 0.40mSv/a	Maximum Hit Rate Specific Energy Hits per annum Cell	Nucleus	Specific Energy Hits /Cell Cycle (30 days) Cell	Nucleus
Radon Betas	0.191					20% of Radon Alpha				
Bronchial Basal		18.0	9	0.0135	0.0541		2.204	0.551	0.181	0.045
Bronchial Secretory		35.4	17.7	0.0035	0.0140		8.526	2.131	0.700	0.175
Bronchiolar Secretory		21.4	10.7	0.0096	0.0383		3.116	0.779	0.256	0.064
U Series	0.267					0.122(UNSCEAR)				
Bronchial Basal		18.0	9	0.0189	0.076		0.645	0.161	0.053	0.013
Bronchial Secretory		35.4	17.7	0.0049	0.020		2.495	0.624	0.205	0.051
Bronchiolar Secretory		21.4	10.7	0.0134	0.054		0.912	0.228	0.075	0.019
Th Series	0.299					0.195(UNSCEAR)				
Bronchial Basal		18.0	9	0.0189	0.076		1.031	0.258	0.085	0.021
Bronchial Secretory		35.4	17.7	0.0049	0.020		3.988	0.997	0.328	0.082
Bronchiolar Secretory		21.4	10.7	0.0134	0.054		1.457	0.364	0.120	0.030
K-40 Terestrial	0.245					0.183(UNSCEAR)				
Bronchial Basal		18.0	9	0.0174	0.069		1.055	0.264	0.087	0.022
Bronchial Secretory		35.4	17.7	0.0045	0.018		4.079	1.020	0.335	0.084
Bronchiolar Secretory		21.4	10.7	0.0123	0.049		1.490	0.373	0.122	0.031
Cosmic	0.060					0.400(UNSCEAR)				
Bronchial Basal		18.0	9	0.0043	0.017		9.412	2.353	0.773	0.193
Bronchial Secretory		35.4	17.7	0.0011	0.004		36.403	9.101	2.990	0.747
Bronchiolar Secretory		21.4	10.7	0.0030	0.012		13.303	3.326	1.093	0.273
Internal	0.245					0.300(UNSCEAR)				
Bronchial Basal		18.0	9	0.0174	0.069		1.729	0.432	0.142	0.035
Bronchial Secretory		35.4	17.7	0.0045	0.018		6.686	1.672	0.549	0.137
Bronchiolar Secretory		21.4	10.7	0.0123	0.049		2.443	0.611	0.201	0.050
Medical	1.52					0.400(UNSCEAR)				
Bronchial Basal		18.0	9	0.1077	0.431		0.372	0.093	0.031	0.008
Bronchial Secretory		35.4	17.7	0.0278	0.111		1.437	0.359	0.118	0.030
Bronchiolar Secretory		21.4	10.7	0.0762	0.305		0.525	0.131	0.043	0.011
Total Specific Energy Hits per Cell Cycle (30 days)										
Bronchial Basal									1.351	0.338
Bronchial Secretory									5.225	1.306
Bronchiolar Secretory									1.909	0.477
Radon Alphas	85					1.248(UNSCEAR)				
Bronchial Basal		18.0	9	6.021	24.083		2.1E-02	5.2E-03	0.002	0.000
Bronchial Secretory		35.4	17.7	1.557	6.227		8.0E-02	2.0E-02	0.007	0.002
Bronchiolar Secretory		21.4	10.7	4.260	17.039		2.9E-02	7.3E-03	0.002	0.001

In Table A2, the annual dose equivalents used are given in Column 6. Columns 7 and 8 provide the total hits per year and finally Columns 9 and 10 provide the total hits per 30 day lung cell cycle for each cell species for each exposure category. At the bottom in Columns (9) and (10), we provide the total low LET radation induced charged particle traversal to each of the lung cell species. Since the bronchial secretory cells are the largest they receive the most hits.

175

Computation of the Variation in Adaptive Response Protection with Variation in Radon Concentration.

As described in the main text, we have estimated the variation in lung cell Specific Energy Hits and the Adaptive Response radio-protection. We have assumed constant representative human exposure values for the cosmic, medical, terrestrial Potassium-40 and Thorium series and internal dose. The radon progeny beta and the terrestrial Uranium dose are assumed to vary with increasing radon concentration as shown in Figure 13.

TABLE A3 – Example Spread Sheet for Calculation of Charged Particle Traversals (Hits) and Poisson Accumulation of Adaptive Response Radio-Protection. This Part for Basel Cell Traversals. Two Other Separate Computations are for Bronchial and Bronchiolar Secretory Cells. Hits and Protection is for 30 Day Mitotic Cycle Exposure.

Radon Bq m-3	Th Series Hits	K-40 Hits	Cosmic Hits	Internal Hits	Medical Hits	Rn Betas Hits	U Series Hits	Radon Hits	Total Basal Hits	AR Poisson Protection
1	0.038	0.043	0.376	0.068	0.015	0.001317	0.006102	0.049383	0.547419	0.683831
2	0.038	0.043	0.376	0.068	0.015	0.002634	0.007088	0.098765	0.549722	0.682833
4	0.038	0.043	0.376	0.068	0.015	0.005267	0.009026	0.197531	4.065412	0.262867
6	0.038	0.043	0.376	0.068	0.015	0.007901	0.010916	0.296296	0.558817	0.678914
8	0.038	0.043	0.376	0.068	0.015	0.010535	0.012758	0.395062	0.563293	0.676998
10	0.038	0.043	0.376	0.068	0.015	0.013169	0.014554	0.493827	0.567722	0.675111
12	0.038	0.043	0.376	0.068	0.015	0.015802	0.016301	0.592593	0.572104	0.673253
14	0.038	0.043	0.376	0.068	0.015	0.018436	0.018002	0.691358	0.576438	0.671422
16	0.038	0.043	0.376	0.068	0.015	0.02107	0.019655	0.790123	0.580725	0.66962
18	0.038	0.043	0.376	0.068	0.015	0.023704	0.02126	0.888889	0.584964	0.667844
20	0.038	0.043	0.376	0.068	0.015	0.026337	0.022818	0.987654	0.589156	0.666097
22	0.038	0.043	0.376	0.068	0.015	0.028971	0.024329	1.08642	0.5933	0.664376
24	0.038	0.043	0.376	0.068	0.015	0.031605	0.025792	1.185185	0.597397	0.662681
26	0.038	0.043	0.376	0.068	0.015	0.034239	0.027208	1.283951	0.601447	0.661014
28	0.038	0.043	0.376	0.068	0.015	0.036872	0.028577	1.382716	0.605449	0.659372
30	0.038	0.043	0.376	0.068	0.015	0.039506	0.029898	1.481481	0.609404	0.657756
32	0.038	0.043	0.376	0.068	0.015	0.04214	0.031171	1.580247	0.613311	0.656166
34	0.038	0.043	0.376	0.068	0.015	0.044774	0.032397	1.679012	0.617171	0.654601
36	0.038	0.043	0.376	0.068	0.015	0.047407	0.033576	1.777778	0.620984	0.653062
38	0.038	0.043	0.376	0.068	0.015	0.050041	0.034708	1.876543	0.624749	0.651547
40	0.038	0.043	0.376	0.068	0.015	0.052675	0.035791	1.975309	0.628466	0.650057
42	0.038	0.043	0.376	0.068	0.015	0.055309	0.036828	2.074074	0.632137	0.648591
44	0.038	0.043	0.376	0.068	0.015	0.057942	0.037817	2.17284	0.63576	0.64715
46	0.038	0.043	0.376	0.068	0.015	0.060576	0.038759	2.271605	0.639335	0.645732
48	0.038	0.043	0.376	0.068	0.015	0.06321	0.039653	2.37037	0.642863	0.644339
50	0.038	0.043	0.376	0.068	0.015	0.065844	0.0405	2.469136	0.646344	0.642969
52	0.038	0.043	0.376	0.068	0.015	0.068477	0.041299	2.567901	0.649777	0.641622
54	0.038	0.043	0.376	0.068	0.015	0.071111	0.042052	2.666667	0.653163	0.640298

PARTS I and II - APPENDIX B

Definitions of Parameters in the Bystander Effect and Adaptive Response Microdose Model, Equation (1) – Leonard (2008)

Adaptive Response Parameters

P_{spo} = Zero priming absorbed dose, spontaneous damage level

RR - Relative Risk - The observed damage level normalized to the spontaneous damage level at zero priming dose (P_{spo}).

$P_{prot-s\infty}$ = The magnitude of the Adaptive Response radio-protection when 100% of the cells are activated and the radio-protection for the spontaneous damage is fully developed.

$P_{prot-pr\infty}$ = The magnitude of the Adaptive Response radio-protection when 100% of the cells are activated and the radio-protection for the primer radiation damage is fully developed.

$PAFs(M,N)$ = The Poisson Accumulation Function as a function of mean number of cell charged particle traversals, M, for the minimum number of Poisson distributed traversals to activate the Adaptive Response radio-protection, N, for the spontaneous damage.

$PAFpr(M,Q)$ = The Poisson Accumulation Function as a function of mean number of cell charged particle traversals, M, for the minimum number of Poisson distributed traversals to activate the Adaptive Response radio-protection, Q, for the primer dose damage.

$RP(t, t_o)$ = The Adaptive Response activation and fading function as a function of time after administering the primer dose and time for the threshold for fading of the AR, t_o. See Equation (5) of Leonard (2007b).

$f(D)$ = The Adaptive Response retention function as the high dose Direct Damage is induced. $f(D)$ = 1.0 as D increases for full retention of the AR radio-protection. $f(D)$ = 0 if the AR is fully dissipated as D increases.

Bystander Effect Parameters

σ = The fraction of cells that are hypersensitive to oncogenic transformation by the bystander signal. For protective Bystander Effects, σ will be negative as a result of the receptor, hypersensitive cells activating protective mechanisms as illustrated in Leonard (2008). For deleterious Bystander Effects, σ will be positive as illustrated by

Brenner et al (2001). k = The number of un-irradiated cells per unit dose (cGy^{-1}) that actually receive a bystander responsive signal.

q = The probability per unit dose (cGy^{-1}) of a cell surviving a single alpha particle traversal of its nucleus.

ξ = The fraction of traversed cells that become inactivated (non-colony forming).

The bystander effect is as a result of a small population of hypersensitive bystander receptor cells such that the [Exp (- ξ q D)] "Depletion" function in Equation (1) characterizes the depletion of these hypersensitive cells by inactivation by Hits from the direct damage. The [1- Exp (- k D)] "Hit probability" function provides the probability per unit dose that at least one cell is directly Hit where as noted k is the number of un-Hit neighbor cells receiving the bystander signal. The combined product [1- Exp (- k D)] [Exp (- ξ q D)] facilitates the dose and specific energy Hits dependence of the total Bystander Damage component.

Direct Damage Parameters

α and β = Linear (cGy^{-1}) and quadratic (cGy^{-2}) Direct Damage coefficients from the conventional Linear-Quadratic dose response formulism (Kellerer and Rossi 1972).

PAF$_D$(M,U) = The Poisson Accumulation Function for low LET adaptive response effects as a function of mean number of cell charged particle traversals, M, for the minimum number (threshold) of Poisson distributed traversals to induce radiation damage (Direct Damage) from the primer dose radiation, U.

N(M,V,SD) = The Normal Distribution accumulation function for the transition threshold between low alpha dose Bystander Damage Region and the high alpha dose Direct Damage Region. V is the mean number of alpha particles to induce the transition and SD is the standard deviation of the Normal Distribution (width at ½ maximum).

INDEX

180

Microdose Model, viii, x, xiv, 11, 22, 25, 39, 42, 47, 59, 62, 64, 66, 67, 68, 70, 73, 76, 78, 80, 115, 124, 126, 128, 131, 140, 145, 151, 168, 188

Mitchel, xi, 9, 68, 75, 77, 143, 147, 148, 154, 158, 170, 171, 173, 174

NCRP, 3, 10, 154

Papworth, ix, 3, 115, 117, 119, 120, 122, 127, 133, 137, 157, 172, 173

protective Bystander, 12, 16, 69, 70, 126, 145, 148, 168, 188

Radiation Effects Research Foundation, 6, 63

RBE, x, 1, 32, 33, 35, 36, 45, 47, 59, 148, 161

Redpath, xi, xiv, 11, 12, 66, 67, 68, 70, 76, 77, 78, 83, 113, 136, 140, 153, 158, 164, 167, 173

specific energy hit, 37, 68, 70, 77

Thompson, 112, 114, 115, 116, 117, 118, 121, 124, 126, 127, 129, 132, 133, 146, 169, 175

Threshold, vii, ix, 3, 4, 7, 10, 36, 39, 61, 111, 113, 114, 116, 117, 121, 127, 128, 130, 131, 132, 134, 146, 150, 151, 152, 156

underground miners, x, 1, 6, 10, 38, 45, 47, 48, 49, 50, 51, 52, 55, 56, 57, 60, 61, 112, 144, 148, 154, 169

UNSCEAR, viii, x, 2, 21, 79, 81, 82, 85, 86, 87, 95, 96, 99, 101, 104, 106, 107, 108, 109, 113, 128, 146, 157, 158, 176, 179, 183, 184

Uranium gamma, xi, 83, 92, 94, 96, 98, 99, 100, 101, 104

USGS, xi, 83, 87, 88, 89, 92, 95, 96, 104, 145

Printed in Great Britain
by Amazon

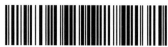

20365652R00112